MAKING GOOD PROGRESS?

The future of Assessment for Learning

Daisy Christodoulou

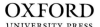

OXFORD
UNIVERSITY PRESS

OXFORD
UNIVERSITY PRESS

Great Clarendon Street, Oxford, OX2 6DP, United Kingdom

Oxford University Press is a department of the University of Oxford.
It furthers the University's objective of excellence in research, scholarship,
and education by publishing worldwide. Oxford is a registered trade mark of
Oxford University Press in the UK and in certain other countries.

ISBN 9780198413608

10 9 8 7 6 5 4 3

Typeset by Carol Hulme

Paper used in the production of this book is a natural, recyclable
product made from wood grown in sustainable forests.

The manufacturing process conforms to the environmental regulations
of the country of origin.

Printed in China by Leo Paper Products Ltd

Acknowledgements

Photographs by Earl Smith: pp.12, 18, 28, 54, 162, 180, 200, 210;
Juice Images/Alamy: p.112; Monkey Business Images/Shutterstock: p.4;
Tyler Olson/Shutterstock p.78; Caiaimage/Chris Ryan/Getty Images: p.138;
Dr Jasper Green: p.120

Other images: Paul Urry/Times Education Supplement: p.114; GL Assessments: p.63

The Publisher would like to thank Larkrise Primary School for permission
to reproduce photographs.

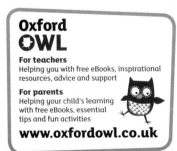

Oxford OWL

For teachers
Helping you with free eBooks, inspirational
resources, advice and support

For parents
Helping your child's learning
with free eBooks, essential
tips and fun activities

www.oxfordowl.co.uk

Table of Contents

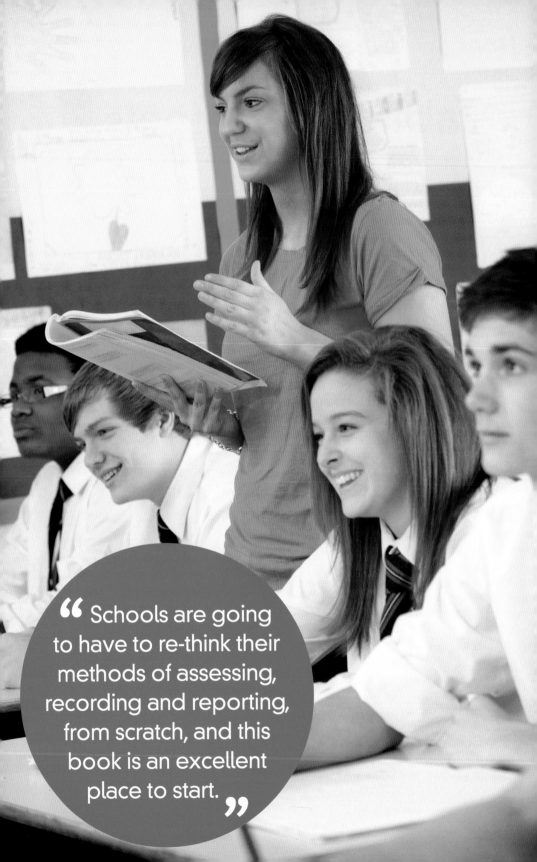

&6 Schools are going to have to re-think their methods of assessing, recording and reporting, from scratch, and this book is an excellent place to start. **99**

Foreword
by Dylan Wiliam

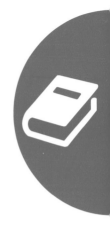

In July 1987, just as schools were breaking up for the summer holidays, the UK government announced its intention to introduce a national curriculum for all schools in England and Wales.[1] Over the summer, working parties were set up to propose what should be in the national curricula for mathematics and science, and, in parallel, the Secretary of State for Education and Science, Kenneth Baker, asked Professor Paul Black to chair the National Curriculum Task Group on Assessment and Testing.

The brief of the Task Group was to advise the Secretary of State for Education and Science, and the Secretary of State for Wales on 'a coherent system of assessment, including testing, to cover the whole period of compulsory schooling'.[2] The Group was specifically asked, in a letter from Baker, to ensure that its recommendations were practicable to implement and cost-effective, but should also:

> take account of the very considerable amount of assessment which is already carried out as a normal part of teaching and learning in our schools, and will recognise that all forms of assessment affect the teaching and learning assessed.

Baker went on to say that he was:

> looking for arrangements which, by supplementing the normal assessments made by teachers in the classroom with simply-administered tests, will offer a clear picture of how pupils, individually and collectively, are faring at each of the age points. Such arrangements should help to promote good teaching.

It seems that Baker had in mind a simple reporting scale whereby each student would get a grade from A to E at the ages of 7, 11, 14 and 16. Such a system of reporting would have the merit of simplicity, but the brief for the Task Group had specifically drawn attention to the fact that assessment affects teaching and learning. The problem with a simple A to E grading system was that a student who got an E at the age of 7 would probably also get an E at the ages of 11, 14, and 16.

At the time, I was working at King's College London, and had been closely involved with a project entitled Graded Assessment in Mathematics (GAIM). The project, directed by Professor Margaret Brown, was developing an assessment system that would meet the needs of all students, rather than just the 60% of students who would, in their final years of compulsory education, be taking courses leading to formal qualifications such as the General Certificate of Education (GCE, or O Level) or the Certificate of Secondary Education (CSE). In particular, we were looking at how to assess students who found learning mathematics difficult in a way that might be motivating rather than alienating.

I had come across the work of Carol Dweck in 1983, when I was teaching at North Westminster Community School, because she had contributed a chapter to a book edited by my headteacher, Michael Marland.[3] Dweck's distinction between 'fixed' and what she called at the time 'incremental' views of intelligence crystallized for me my concerns with many assessment models. If a student keeps on getting a C, then she is likely to come to think of herself as a C student. If the student keeps on making progress, the student is more likely to believe that intelligence is malleable—by working, you're getting smarter.

The idea of age-independent levels of achievement had been a strong feature of the Secondary Mathematics Individualised Learning Experiment (SMILE)[4] mathematics scheme that I had introduced at North Westminster Community School and so, when we were looking at reporting achievement in the GAIM project we tried to do the same thing—put all students on the same ladder, and ensure that all students experience progression.

Because we were focusing on the 13 to 16 age range, and in particular, low achievers within that age range, we felt that each student would need to achieve at least one level every year for the effects to be motivating. By use of archives of data from research projects such as Concepts in Secondary Mathematics and Science[5], and the reports of the Assessment of Performance Unit[6], Alice Onion—another researcher on the GAIM project—and I realized that to give every student in the 13-16 age range a reasonable chance of achieving one level every year, 13 to 15 levels of achievement would be needed.

Brown presented these ideas to the Task Group in the Autumn of 1987, and at one point, one of the group members asked how many additional levels would be needed to cover the primary age-range. Brown's estimate was that five additional levels would be needed. In other words, to give each student a reasonable chance of achieving one level a year, 20 levels would be needed.

While meaningfully identifying 20 levels of achievement might be possible in mathematics and science, no-one thought it would be possible in history or

English. The proposal of the Task Group was therefore to have a system of ten levels, designed so that the average student would achieve one level every two years. This made a lot of sense, because the intention was that student achievement would be reported only at the end of a key stage, so most students would experience progression in their reported level each time their achievement was reported.

Some years later, it was decided that the grades of the newly created General Certificate of Secondary Education (GCSE), which resulted from combining the Ordinary level of the GCE examinations with CSE, should continue to be used for the end of key stage 4, so the national curriculum assessment system was trimmed back to eight levels, covering students from 7 to 14.

This detail is important because it is often alleged that the ten (and later, eight) levels of the national curriculum assessment system were arbitrary, whereas the system was designed on the best research we had on student progression, and on the effects of grades and scores on student learning.

Over the following quarter century, the national curriculum was reviewed and updated many times, and on a number of occasions, the idea of age-independent levels of achievement was challenged. In his final report on the 1993 review of the national curriculum and its assessment, Sir Ron Dearing wrote: 'I am not convinced that the end of key stage scale provides a demonstrably better way to assess pupil achievement'[7] and the ten-level model survived.

Had schools continued to report national curriculum levels to parents at the end of each key stage (which is all they were ever required to do) then everything would have been fine. But over the succeeding years, schools started reporting levels at the end of every year, at the end of each term, and then, most bizarrely of all, schools started putting levels on individual pieces of work, displaying a staggering level of assessment illiteracy, since the levels were meant to be summaries of a student's achievement across an entire key stage. Even worse, inspectors from the Office for Standards in Education, Children's Services and Skills (Ofsted) would ask students what levels they were working at, and so, predictably, schools ensured that their students were able to respond with an appropriate number.

That is why, when, in 2010, I was appointed as a member of an 'Expert Panel' to advise Michael Gove, then Secretary of State for Education, on changes to the national curriculum and its assessment, I recommended that national curriculum levels should be abolished. I did so with no enthusiasm. I had always supported the idea of age-independent levels of achievement. I was convinced that such a system was more compatible with the idea of what Dweck now calls a 'growth mindset' and anything else would undermine efforts by schools to persuade students that 'Smart is not something that you just are, smart is something that you can get.'[8] But what was happening in schools was so antithetical to good teaching, I thought whatever benefits national curriculum levels might bring were more than out-weighed by the negative consequences.

So, national curriculum levels have gone, and they will not be replaced. This has, predictably, been very disorientating for a lot of people, since many teachers and parents have known nothing else. But it is important to realize that the abolition of national curriculum levels represents an extraordinary opportunity for schools. It means that school inspectors can no longer ask how many students are making 'three levels of progress' or other equally fatuous questions. Schools will still need to ensure that they have good ways of finding out whether their students are making progress. When Ofsted inspectors ask, 'How do you know your students are making progress?' schools had better have a good answer to that question. But they are now free to choose ways of monitoring student progress that work best for them.

Most importantly, schools can develop assessment systems that take into account what we know about how learning takes place, and that is why this book by Daisy Christodoulou is so timely. As she makes clear, most school assessment systems rest on a profound fallacy—that the best way to monitor progress in learning is to judge progress by how far the student falls short of the level of performance that will be expected at the end of the learning.

The logic is attractive, but wrong. Over hundreds of years, we have learned that practising scales when learning a musical instrument is helpful even if you will never actually play a scale in playing a piece of music. Sports coaches know the value of drills even though they seem remote from the kinds of skills that will be needed in competition. And in the same way, research is now demonstrating how to apply these lessons in academic learning.

For twenty years, I have been puzzling about the relationship between formative and summative functions of assessment. My initial instinct was that they could and should be integrated. After all, any assessment is just an attempt to determine what a student can do, and if the same assessments can serve both functions, then the time needed for assessment is reduced, leaving more time for teaching and learning. However in this wide-ranging and important book Christodoulou has, to my mind, convincingly demonstrated that while the formative and summative uses of assessments have to co-exist, they must also be kept apart. Record-keeping that details a student's progress towards test and examination success is unlikely to help achieve that success. Schools are going to have to re-think their methods of assessing, recording, and reporting, from scratch, and this book is an excellent place to start.

Notes

1 Department of Education and Science, & Welsh Office, 1987. *The National Curriculum 5-16: a consultation document*. London, UK: Department of Education and Science <http://www.educationengland.org.uk/documents/des/nc-consultation.html>
   The above consultation resulted in the publication of the following report: National Curriculum Task Group on Assessment and Testing. 1988. *A report*. London, UK: Department of Education and Science. <http://www.educationengland.org.uk/documents/pdfs/1988-TGAT-report.pdf>

2 National Curriculum Task Group on Assessment and Testing. 1988. *A report: Appendix B* p.2 <http://www.kcl.ac.uk/sspp/departments/education/research/Research-Centres/crestem/Research/Current-Projects/assessment/tgatappen.pdf>

3 Licht, B. G., & Dweck, C. S., 1983. Sex differences in achievement orientations: Consequences for academic choices and attainments. In M. Marland (Ed.), *Sex differentiation and schooling* (pp. 72-97). London, UK: Hodder & Stoughton.

4 SMILE stood, originally, for the Secondary Mathematics Individualized Learning Experiment. Over the years this has been the subject of some revisionism, with claims that it stood for Secondary Mathematics Individualized Learning Experience, or even just Secondary Mathematics Individualized LEarning.

5 Hart, K.M., 1980. *Secondary School Children's Understanding of Mathematics*. A Report of the Mathematics Component of the Concepts in Secondary Mathematics and Science Programme.
   See also: Hart, K. M. (Ed.), 1981. *Children's understanding of mathematics: 11-16*. London, UK: John Murray

6 For example: Foxman, D. D., Badger, M. E., Martini, R. M., & Mitchell, P., 1981. *Mathematical development: secondary survey report no 2*. London, UK: Her Majesty's Stationery Office (HMSO).
   Foxman, D. D., Cresswell, M. J., & Badger, M. E., 1981. *Mathematical development: primary survey report no 2*. London, UK: HMSO.
   Foxman, D. D., Cresswell, M. J., Ward, M., Badger, M. E., Tuson, J. A, & Bloomfield, B. A, 1980. *Mathematical development: primary survey report no 1*. London, UK: HMSO.
   Foxman, D. D., Martini, R. M., & Mitchell, P., 1982. *Mathematical development: secondary survey report no 3*. London, UK: HMSO.
   Foxman, D. D., Martini, R. M., Tuson, J. A, & Cresswell, M. J., 1980. *Mathematical development: secondary survey report no 1*. London, UK: HMSO.
   Foxman, D. D., Ruddock, G. J., Badger, M. E., & Martini, R. M., 1982. *Mathematical development: primary survey report no 3*. London, UK: HMSO.

7 Dearing, R, 1994. *The National Curriculum and its assessment: Final report*. London, UK: School Curriculum and Assessment Authority p.70

8 Howard, J., 1991. *Getting smart: the social construction of intelligence*. Waltham, MA: Efficacy Institute p.7

About the author

Daisy Christodoulou is the Head of Assessment at Ark Schools, where she works on assessment reform, replacements for National Curriculum levels and readiness for new national exams. Previously, she was Research and Development Manager at Ark, working closely on curriculum reform in secondary English.

Before that, she trained as a secondary English teacher through the Teach First programme and taught in two London comprehensives. Her book, *Seven Myths About Education*, was published in March 2014. She has been part of government commissions on the future of teacher training and assessment.

Acknowledgements

Many people helped me to write this book.

Dylan Wiliam, Maria Egan, Greg Ashman, Heather Fearn, Joe Kirby, Daniel Willingham, Michelle Major, Robert Peal, Michael Slavinsky and Daniel Lavipour all offered helpful comments on early drafts. At Ark schools, I have been supported, encouraged and inspired by many people and am particularly grateful to Brian Sims, Rebecca Curtis, Venessa Willms, Veronica Lloyd-Richards, Rich Davies, Amy McJennett, Nick Wallace, Jasper Green and Amanda Spielman.

Any mistakes that remain are, of course, my own responsibility.

We have lost the tools of learning--the axe and the wedge, the hammer and the saw, the chisel and the plane-- that were so adaptable to all tasks. Instead of them, we have merely a set of complicated jigs, each of which will do but one task and no more, and in using which eye and hand receive no training, so that no man ever sees the work as a whole or "looks to the end of the work".

Dorothy L. Sayers, *The Lost Tools of Learning*

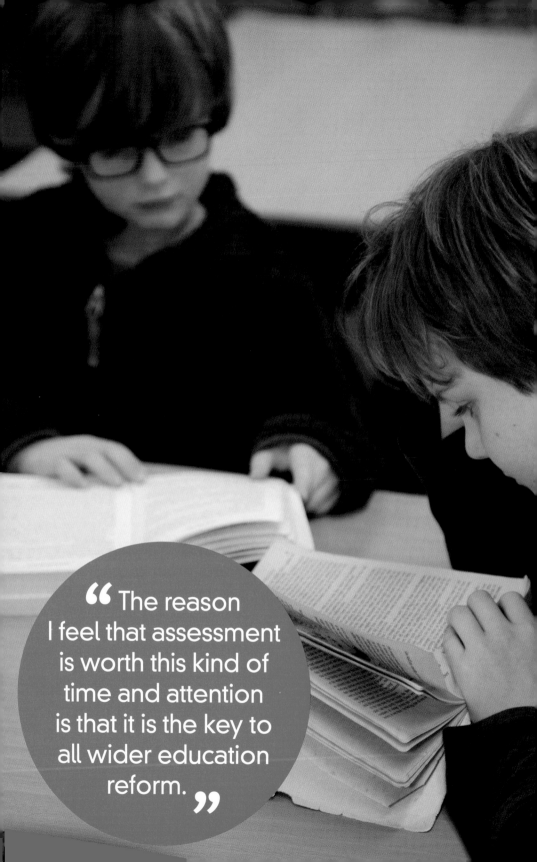

> **"** The reason I feel that assessment is worth this kind of time and attention is that it is the key to all wider education reform. **"**

Introduction

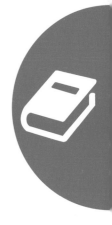

In my previous book, *Seven Myths About Education*, I argued that the dominant educational orthodoxy about how we should teach and learn was based on flimsy foundations. In the UK, teacher training courses and the Office for Standards in Education, Children's Services and Skills (Ofsted) encouraged independent project-based learning, promoted the teaching of transferable skills, and made bold claims about how the Internet could replace memory. In actual fact, the scientific evidence showed that pupils learn best with direct instruction, that to develop skill we need to remember large bodies of knowledge, and that independent projects overwhelm our limited working memories. This book has its origins in two common responses to these arguments: one negative, one positive.

The negative response was from people who argued that there was, in fact, a lot more direct instruction of knowledge in English schools than I'd suggested, and that good evidence for this was the fact that schools were so much more exam-focussed than they used to be.[1-2] This worried me because it suggested that for many people, direct instruction of knowledge and 'teaching to the test' – or teaching with a primary focus on preparing for national tests – were synonymous. In fact, I felt that the two were not similar at all. Many popular exam-preparation activities were directly opposed to what I was recommending and, indeed, directly opposed to any conception of good education. Advice on exam preparation was all about drilling pupils in the marks-to-minute ratio of exam papers and the key phrases examiners expected to see. Textbooks gave almost as much space to the intricacies of a particular exam board's style of questions as they did to the actual content of the course.[3] I was in favour of lots of practice and repetition, but of powerful knowledge that would be of value to pupils for the rest of their life, not exam shortcuts. So, the first aim of this book is to look at the differences between education that is focussed only on exam success, and education that is focussed on developing enduring and valuable knowledge and skills.

The positive response came from people who were keen to implement some of these ideas in their classroom or school, but who found that one of the main obstacles was assessment. How was it possible to implement a knowledge-rich curriculum when national exams required something quite different? Ofsted wanted to see progress in every lesson: how would that work if a lesson was based around practice and consolidation of content that had been learned before? Then there were National Curriculum levels, the government's national assessment system in England which was used in the classroom and for external tests. When *Seven Myths About Education* was first published in 2013, they had just been abolished and schools were designing their replacements for them. The need for a new assessment system prompted me and many other teachers to think about the relationship between the curriculum, assessment and pedagogy. What would be the best kind of assessment system that could help promote evidence-based teaching practices? What were the flaws with levels that we should seek to avoid with any new system? Over the past three years, I have spent a lot of time thinking about these questions: first as a teacher at Pimlico Academy, a secondary school in London, and now as Head of Assessment at Ark Schools, a network of 35 primary and secondary academy schools in England. The second aim of this book is to attempt to answer these questions.

I start in Chapters 1 and 2 by looking at Assessment for Learning (AfL). AfL was one of the most promising educational innovations of the past few decades, yet it failed to improve education in the way many had hoped. Although its aim was to use assessment to help pupils learn, rather than to produce grades, in the worst cases it actually ended up encouraging 'teaching to the test' and over-frequent grading. I argue that this was because, in practice, the value of exam tasks was overestimated, and other types of assessment were undervalued. Counter-intuitively, I felt that this kind of teaching to the test was more likely to be caused by a belief in independent and project-based learning than it was by a belief in direct knowledge instruction. Direct instruction involves breaking things down: taking a complex skill, breaking it into its smallest parts and teaching those small parts. This results in lessons and activities that look very different to the activities on the final exam paper. By contrast, project-based learning suggests that the best way for pupils to learn is to practise authentic tasks. Although at first sight such projects seem very different from exams, in practice there are some similarities, as exam tasks often try to be authentic too. A project-based approach to learning might require pupils to write a letter to their local councillor about recycling, for example, and similar tasks can be found in many exams.

In Chapter 3, I look at what assessment theory has to say about the relationship between tests and learning. Can exam tasks be used to help learning? To what extent can the same task be used both to give pupils a grade, and to give them useful feedback? How valid and reliable are the assessments which try to do both?

In Chapters 4 and 5, I analyse two popular in-school assessment systems: descriptor-based systems, which award a grade by judging work against descriptors, and exam-based systems, which award a grade based on exam performance. How valid and reliable are each of these systems?

In the final four chapters, I put forward some alternative ways of assessing. In Chapter 6, I discuss the importance of an accurate model of progression and different ways of communicating such a model. In Chapter 7, I look at the principles which should guide formative assessments. In Chapter 8, I look at the principles which should guide summative assessments. Finally, in Chapter 9, I give a brief explanation of how to integrate various different assessments into one system.

The reason I feel that assessment is worth this kind of time and attention is that it is the key to all wider educational reform. I have realised that, in practice, any attempt to change curriculum or pedagogy also requires a change in assessment. Often, curriculum statements can be vague and capable of being interpreted in many different ways; it is through the creation of assessments that their actual meaning is defined. Or, as educationalist Dylan Wiliam says, 'assessments operationalise constructs'.[4] So, whilst assessment is only one part of the education debate, it is a part with enormous practical importance. My hope, therefore, is that better ideas about assessment can be the means of making real improvements in learning.

Notes

1 See, for example: BBC Radio Four Current Affairs, 2012. School of hard facts [transcript of a recorded documentary originally broadcast on 22 October 2012] <http://news.bbc.co.uk/1/shared/spl/hi/programmes/analysis/transcripts/221012.pdf> accessed 20 August 2016

2 See, for example: Sherrington, T., 2013. A Perspective on Seven Myths. *headguruteacher*, 5 August [Blog] <https://headguruteacher.com/2013/08/05/a-perspective-on-seven-myths/> accessed 20 August 2016

3 See, for example: Oates, T., 2014. *Why textbooks count: A policy paper*. Cambridge: University of Cambridge Local Examinations Syndicate, pp.4–5

4 Wiliam, D., 2010. What counts as evidence of educational achievement? The role of constructs in the pursuit of equity in assessment. In Luke, A., Green, J. and Kelly, G., eds. *What counts as evidence in educational settings? Rethinking equity, diversity and reform in the 21st century*. Washington: American Educational Research Association, pp.254–284

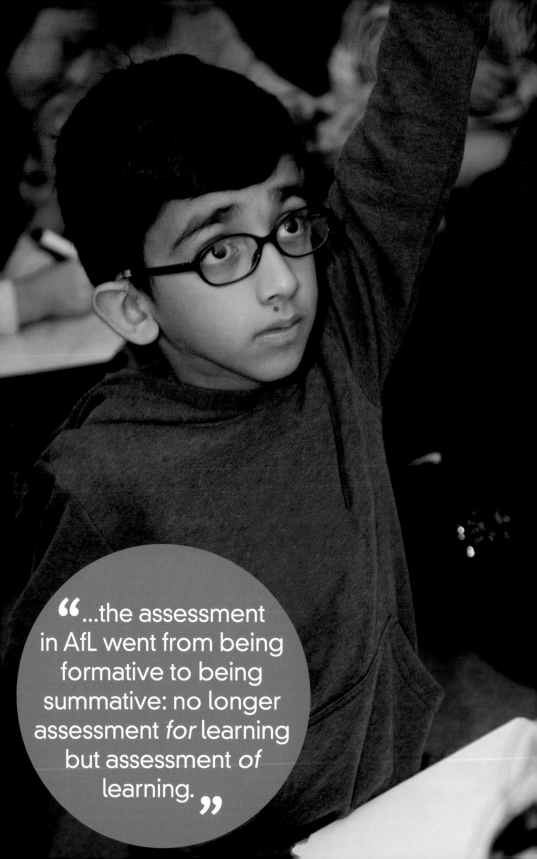

"...the assessment in AfL went from being formative to being summative: no longer assessment *for* learning but assessment *of* learning."

Why didn't Assessment for Learning transform our schools?

1

One of the most promising educational innovations of the last few decades was Assessment for Learning (AfL). AfL, or formative assessment, has been defined by Wiliam as when teachers 'use evidence of student learning to adapt teaching and learning, or instruction, to meet student needs.'[1] The concept of formative assessment was developed and popularised by Dylan Wiliam and Paul Black, two well-respected education professors. It was based on decades of solid research showing that giving feedback to pupils dramatically improved their progress.[2] Unusually, the idea was met with little opposition, and was in fact welcomed by both government and teachers. As Robert Coe, Professor of Education, argues, '[AfL] became the focus of national policy, widely endorsed by teachers and supported by extensive government training, following the publication of Black and Wiliam's (1998) *Inside the Black Box*... It is now a rare thing, in my experience, to meet any teacher in any school in England who would not claim to be doing Assessment for Learning.'[3] The 2013 Teaching and Learning International Survey (TALIS) confirms Coe's experience: in comparison to other countries, teachers in England give a lot of oral and written feedback to pupils.[4]

As Coe also goes on to argue, despite this propitious beginning, AfL has not had the kind of success you might expect:

> ...During the fifteen years of this intensive intervention to promote AfL, despite its near universal adoption and strong research evidence of substantial impact on attainment, there has been no (or at best limited) effect on learning outcomes nationally.
>
> Coe, R., *Improving Education: A triumph of hope over experience*, p.10

Nor is Coe alone in claiming this. Wiliam and Black themselves have spoken of their disappointment in the way that the policy has been implemented: in 2012, Wiliam said that 'there are very few schools where all the principles of AfL, as I understand them, are being implemented effectively.'[5] Wiliam also noted that in many cases, whilst teachers had followed his advice in *Inside the Black Box* and replaced grades with comments, the comments they were providing were not necessarily that helpful – or that formative:

> Typically, the feedback would focus on what was deficient about the work submitted, which the students were not able to resubmit, rather than on what to do to improve their future learning...I remember talking to a middle school student who was looking at the feedback his teacher had given him on a science assignment. The teacher had written, "You need to be more systematic in planning your scientific inquiries." I asked the student what that meant to him, and he said, "I don't know. If I knew how to be more systematic, I would have been more systematic the first time." This kind of feedback is accurate—it is describing what needs to happen—but it is not helpful because the learner does not know how to use the feedback to improve. It is rather like telling an unsuccessful comedian to be funnier— accurate, but not particularly helpful, advice.
>
> Wiliam, D., *Embedded formative assessment*, p.120

Wiliam also said that, 'We have (Department for Education officials) saying: "We tried AfL and it didn't work." But that's because (they) didn't try the AfL that does work.'[5] How has this happened? Why did a policy with so much academic, government and grass-roots support end up being implemented so badly?

One possible explanation is that government support for the policy was, in fact, counter-productive. When government get their hands on anything involving the word 'assessment', they want it to be about high-stakes monitoring and tracking, not low-stakes diagnostics. That is, the involvement of government in AfL meant that the assessment in AfL went from being formative to being summative: no longer assessment *for* learning but assessment *of* learning. The difference may be just one preposition, but it is profound. When assessment is formative, the aim is to reveal pupils' weaknesses so the teacher can act on them. When assessment is summative, the aim is to give pupils a final grade, and so there can be pressure to try to conceal and gloss over misunderstandings. Indeed, formative assessment is so different from summative assessment that Wiliam has said that he wished he had called AfL 'responsive teaching', rather than using the word assessment.[6] He has also said that, 'The problem is that government told schools that it was all about monitoring pupils' progress; it wasn't about pupils becoming owners of their own learning.'[5] AfL is not just about teachers being responsive; it is also about pupils responding to information about their progress.

The pressures placed on assessment have almost certainly, therefore, played a part in the failure of AfL. Internationally, the Organisation for Ecomonic Co-operation and Development (OECD) has shown that all assessment systems struggle with the competing formative and summative functions of assessment.[7] In England, this problem is exacerbated by the pressures of a high-stakes accountability system. Schools are judged by how well their pupils perform on summative terminal exams such as Key Stage 2 national tests (commonly known as SATs), General Certificate of Secondary Education tests (GCSEs) and General Certificate of Education Advanced Level tests (A levels). Not only that, but schools are also judged by the performance of their pupils in interim teacher assessments. When Ofsted inspect a school, they don't just look at the most recent national results. They also want to see the most recent teacher assessment data for pupils.[8] Therefore, there is clearly a great deal of pressure on these sets of data. Schools might want to set up internal assessment systems that aim to diagnose weakness, but the fact that the data in the system will be used by Ofsted to judge a school will make that much less likely.

Whilst there is undoubtedly some truth to this explanation, I do not think it accounts for the whole problem. Like many explanations which lay the blame at the door of Ofsted or government, it prompts another question: why did Ofsted and government distort AfL in this way? In this case, I think that the problems surrounding the implementation of AfL are the result of even more fundamental debates about the best methods of education.

In England, there is some consensus around the final aims of education. Literacy and numeracy are clearly vital skills which pupils need to be able to function in a modern economy and society. As well as these, developing skills such as critical thinking and problem solving are often agreed to be important aims of a modern education. Few people would be happy with an education which churned out pupils capable of reading basic texts and doing basic sums, but unable to think critically and creatively about problems they haven't seen before. Similarly, few would defend a system that ignored the basics of literacy and numeracy. The National Curriculum in England has been changed and revised since it was introduced almost thirty years ago, but its various versions stress the importance of the skills listed earlier.[9] However, whilst there may be some agreement on these aims, there is more controversy regarding the best methods which will achieve them. We will explore these debates in more detail in the next chapter. For now, it is possible to summarise two broad approaches to developing such skills.

Teaching skills directly – the generic-skill method

One approach, which we will call a generic-skill method, is to teach a skill directly. If you want pupils to learn how to read, get them to read real books. If you want them to be good at solving maths problems, get them to solve maths problems. If you want them to think critically, set up activities and tasks that will give them the opportunity to think critically. In practice, such approaches might involve an element of project-based learning, where lessons are organised around skills such as problem solving, communication or critical thinking, rather than subject categories. So, for example, pupils might carry out a project where they work out the best place to site a new airport, or one where they design a leaflet to help guide people around a local museum. The idea is that if pupils work on solving problems which are more like the ones they might face in real life, this will help them to get better at solving such problems.

Teaching skills indirectly – the deliberate-practice method

An alternative approach, which we'll call the deliberate-practice method, argues that the best way to impart such skills is to teach them more indirectly. Whilst skills such as literacy, numeracy, problem solving and critical thinking are still the end point of education, this does not mean that pupils always need to be practising such skills in their final form. Instead, the role of the teacher, and indeed the various parts of the education system, should be to break down such skills into their component parts and to teach those instead. This means that lessons may look very different from the final skill they are hoping to instil. For example, a lesson which aims to teach pupils reading may involve pupils learning letter-sound correspondences. A lesson with the ultimate aim of teaching pupils to solve maths problems may involve memorising times tables. The idea here is that the best way to develop skills may not always look like the skill itself.

The importance of debate about methods

These debates about educational methods are absolutely crucial to debates around formative assessment, because formative assessment is all about methods, whereas summative assessment is about aims. Or, to put it another way, different approaches to developing skill don't necessarily affect the assessment *of* learning. Because the outcome is less disputed than the method, the final assessment of learning won't look particularly different. We might agree, for example, that pupils should be able to write an essay about the causes of the First World War by the end of their time in school, perform a successful science experiment, talk intelligently about a character's motivation in *Macbeth*, or work out the standard deviation of a set of data.

Different interpretations of how we acquire skill really do affect assessment *for* learning. This is because these different interpretations are all about the *method* of acquiring skill. Assessment for learning is also all about the method, and the process, of acquiring skill. If we return to our earlier example, we may agree that pupils should be able to write an essay about the causes of the First World War by the end of their time in school, but we may differ on the process and the methods that will lead to them being able to write that essay. This will, therefore, fundamentally affect the assessment for learning that takes place as a part of this process.

If you subscribe to the generic-skill method, then very similar tasks can be used for assessment of learning and assessment for learning. The final assessment of learning should be the pattern for all teaching and all formative assessment. If the final assessment is to write an essay about the causes of the First World War, then the formative assessment should also be to write an essay about the causes of the First World War, or perhaps to write a shorter version of the essay, or an essay about a related issue. This essay would then be marked and given feedback which would inform the pupil's next attempt at the essay. In this model, the assessment for learning tasks are very similar to the assessment of learning tasks. There are just more of them and they receive feedback. The result of this model is to do lots of tasks which have been designed to produce summative information but to add formative feedback to them.

On the other hand, if you believe that the methods that should be used to acquire skill are different from the skill itself (the deliberate-practice method), then assessment for learning looks completely different to assessment of learning. In this case, the terminal assessment is the end goal but the teacher or the curriculum designer must carefully break down that end goal into its constituent parts. So, if the aim is to get pupils to write an essay about the causes of the First World War, then formative assessments will consist of a range of different assessments which may look nothing like the final assessment. For example, formative assessments for this task may consist of short-answer questions that respond to a textbook article, multiple-choice questions about the causes of the war, activities that place key events in the build-up to the war in order, spelling tests on the key figures of the era, and narrative descriptions of key events. In this model, pupils may not even begin to write analytical prose until relatively late in the unit of work. In some units of work, they may never write any analytical prose, but the unit will still help to develop their skills of analysis by developing the skills and knowledge which underpin such analysis. With this model, most of the activities pupils do will not look like the final assessment, but the assumption is that these tasks will help pupils to do better on the final assessment.

One interesting implication of these different methods is that the generic-skill method is more likely to end up focusing narrowly on exam tasks because its model of skill acquisition suggests that practising a complex skill leads one to become better at it. The argument of this book is that assessment for learning became excessively focused on exam tasks not just because of the pressures of accountability, but because the dominant theory of how we acquire skill suggested that was the best thing to do. The argument of this book is also that this dominant theory of skill acquisition is flawed. Not only has this model led to a narrow focus on exam tasks, it has also been ineffective at developing the skills that are its aim.

Because formative assessment is about methods, these debates about how pupils develop skill are crucial. It's therefore worthwhile considering the research around these different methods of skill development in more detail, which we will do in the next chapter.

Notes

1 Wiliam, D., 2009. *Assessment for learning: What, why and how*. London: Institute of Education, University of London

2 Black, P. and Wiliam, D., 1998. *Inside the black box: Raising standards through classroom assessment*. London: King's College

3 Coe, R., 2013. *Improving Education: A triumph of hope over experience*. Durham: Centre for Evaluation and Monitoring, Durham University, p.10

4 Micklewright, J., Jerrim, J., Vignoles, A., Jenkins, A., Allen, R., Ilie, S., Bellarbre, E., Barrera, F. and Hein, C., 2014. *Teachers in England's Secondary Schools: Evidence from TALIS 2013*. London: Institute of Education, University of London, p.154

5 Quoted in Stewart, W., 2012. Think you've implemented Assessment for Learning?. *Times Educational Supplement*, 13 July <https://www.tes.com/article.aspx?storycode=6261847> accessed 6 November 2016

6 Wiliam, D., 2013. Example of really big mistake: calling formative assessment formative assessment rather than something like "responsive teaching" [Twitter] 23 October <https://twitter.com/dylanwiliam/status/393045049337847808> accessed 6 November 2016

7 Organisation for Economic Co-operation and Development (OECD), 2013. *Synergies for Better Learning: An International Perspective on Evaluation and Assessment*. Paris: OECD publishing

8 Ofsted, August 2015. *School inspection handbook: Handbook for inspecting schools in England under section 5 of the Education Act 2005*, p.12

9 For example, whilst the 2007 and 2013 versions of the National Curriculum had significant differences, in many ways the aims were quite similar: the 2007 English curriculum says that pupils should 'develop skills in speaking, listening, reading and writing that they will need to participate in society and employment… learn to express themselves creatively and imaginatively and to communicate with others confidently and effectively… learn to become enthusiastic and critical readers of stories, poetry and drama as well as non-fiction and media texts, gaining access to the pleasure and world of knowledge that reading offers'. The 2013 version says that pupils should learn 'to speak and write fluently so that they can communicate their ideas and emotions to others and through their reading and listening, others can communicate with them…. to develop their love of literature through widespread reading for enjoyment… write clearly, accurately and coherently, adapting their language and style in and for a range of contexts, purposes and audiences'. *The National Curriculum 2007*, p.61 <http://webarchive.nationalarchives.gov.uk/20100202100434/http://curriculum.qcda.gov.uk/uploads/QCA-07-3332-pEnglish3_tcm8-399.pdf>; *National curriculum in England: English programmes of study*, 2013, p.2 <https://www.gov.uk/government/uploads/system/uploads/attachment_data/file/244215/SECONDARY_national_curriculum_-_English2.pdf> accessed 6 November 2016

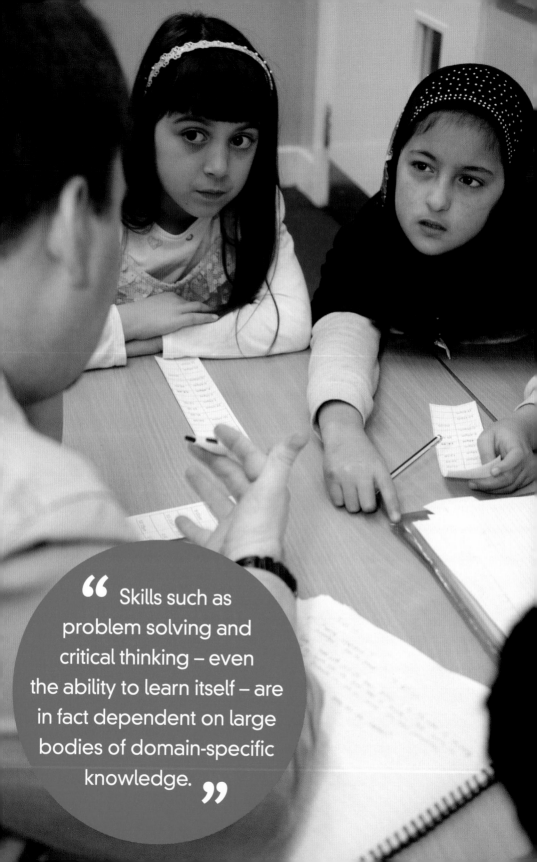

" Skills such as problem solving and critical thinking – even the ability to learn itself – are in fact dependent on large bodies of domain-specific knowledge. **"**

Curriculum aims and teaching methods

In this chapter, we will consider the differences between two methods of skill acquisition (the generic-skill method and the deliberate-practice method) in a bit more detail and look at some examples of how such models work in the classroom.

First, the generic-skill method. As we've seen, this approach suggests that the best way to learn a skill is to practise the skill in a form close to its final version. Not only that, but it suggests that these kinds of skills are generic and transferable across different domains so what matters most is practising the skill: the content can be interchangeable. In the words of Guy Claxton, Professor of Education, 'the generic ability to learn has no use-by date at all', so this generic ability is the one we should teach.[1] Claxton also argues that we need to make sure pupils develop important mental muscle groups:

> *Which mental muscle groups are specifically exercised by maths, or history or music? Can favourite topics defend their place if looked at in this light?*
>
> Claxton, G., *Learning to learn: A key goal in a 21st century curriculum*

The 'mental muscles' analogy implies that skills are transferable and teachable: just as you can train a real muscle to improve its generic performance, so schools should focus on training pupils' mental muscles so they can perform better at learning, problem solving and critical thinking.

In practice, perhaps the purest application of the generic-skill method is the project-based approach, where lessons are organised around skills and cross-curricular projects rather than around subjects. For example, the Royal Society for the Encouragement of Arts, Manufactures and Commerce (RSA) Opening Minds curriculum is organised around five key skills, or competences, rather than subjects. The five skills are: citizenship, learning, managing information, relating to people, and managing situations.[2] In practice, this often means that individual lessons are organised around projects and topics rather than subjects. One school organised its Opening Minds lessons around the following projects: *Where's the Evidence?*; *Let's Get Organised*; *Changes*; *One to One*; *Fit and Healthy*; *Communities*.[3] Another school did something similar on the grounds that it would: 'help to develop transferable skills and competences such as literacy, numeracy and ICT in the Key Stage 3 curriculum' and 'embed Learning to Learn and Emotional Intelligence into the curriculum.'[4]

> *The OM [Opening Minds] projects have been mapped against the National Curriculum but with a focus on the skills rather than the content. It is evident when the National Curriculum is scrutinised in this way that there is much similarity in subject requirements, e.g. all subject areas require students to evaluate, describe, explain etc. Students need these and many other strategies to be successful in life.*
>
> Boyle, H., *Opening Minds*, p.3

Ofsted have praised similar approaches in their publications:

During Year 7, every pupil completed six projects, each lasting half a term, on the themes of 'journeys', 'identity', 'positive images', 'art attack', 'survival' and 'the power and the glory'. These drew on geography, history, religious education, dance, drama, art, and personal, social and health education. The pupils were able to assess their development against defined competencies, weekly or in individual lessons. As a result, they gained an understanding of their strengths and weaknesses which provided a powerful stimulus to learning and raising standards.

Ofsted, *Curriculum innovation in schools*, pp.9–10

The implication here is that as it is the skill that matters, the content can be interchangeable. One obvious implication of this, as we have seen, is to organise the curriculum around projects which promote the direct teaching of such transferable skills. However, even if one does not adopt a fully project-based curriculum structure, it is still possible to introduce this kind of generic-skill approach into a subject-based curriculum, and this approach, too, has been popular. The following English lesson, praised in an Ofsted report, is designed to get pupils to learn by doing a real-life project of the type they might encounter in the workplace:

A group of more able students was producing a school radio programme. The students had decided to create a soap opera, using a range of characters to explore issues of interest to a teenage audience. It was to be presented as part of the daily broadcasts for students. The inspector observed a writers' meeting, where students (supported by the teacher) worked on a script for one of the programmes. An earlier version of the script had been presented to members of the school's pastoral team who had suggested changes. As a result, members of the writing team worked closely together to introduce some new elements to the script. The meeting was a remarkably successful and realistic one, taking on all the elements of the kind of writers' meeting that you might get as part of a real TV or radio soap opera. One of the students described it as 'creative writing mixed with reality'. There was a very open discussion, with students making suggestions and editing as they worked. The inspector noted that the normal roles of teacher and learner appeared to have merged.

Ofsted, *Moving English forward: Action to raise standards in English,* pp.52–53

Another example from a science lesson shows pupils working independently on a real-life project:

Year 8 students were completing a unit of work on acids and alkalis that had involved them in research on the effect of acid rain on limestone. They had worked in groups to generate their own questions to pursue. Many of them had taken the time to form hypotheses and had planned and carried out their own practical work. The students had presented the outcomes of their research to the class in the form of high-quality PowerPoint presentations. Discussion with the students showed how varied these presentations were.

Ofsted, *Successful science:*
An evaluation of science education in England 2007–2010, pp.17–18

For evidence of the popularity and institutional dominance of this approach, see my previous book, *Seven Myths About Education.* As part of the research for this book, I collected examples of 228 lessons that were praised by Ofsted in their publications from 2010–12, and found that many of them recommended this generic-skill method of education.[5]

With all of these approaches, the suggestion is that skills such as problem solving and critical thinking are discrete and teachable. It's assumed that pupils can learn such skills directly and that they can transfer such skills across different tasks and content areas. In order to get better at problem solving, solve problems. In order to get better at thinking critically, practise thinking critically. Once pupils have acquired this generic set of skills, they will be able to apply them in later life to whatever set of problems they encounter.

Skill isn't generic

Such ideas and practices have a great deal of support within education, but they are based on an understanding of skill which doesn't take into account research from the last fifty years about how we think and solve problems. These kinds of generic-skill lessons are not actually effective at instilling the skills they claim to because they misinterpret skill as something that is generic when, in fact, skill is specific. As we will see, research from the field of cognitive psychology shows that the kinds of skills and competences listed in the previous paragraph are not, in fact, separate and discrete abilities which can be taught generically and transferred easily. Skills such as problem solving and critical thinking – even the ability to learn itself – are in fact dependent on large bodies of domain-specific knowledge, and they are not easily transferable to different domains.

Some of the classic research on this point was carried out with chess players. Adriaan de Groot, a Dutch psychologist, researcher and chess master, carried out some of the pioneering studies in the 1940s.[6] Herbert Simon, an American Nobel Laureate, followed up on these studies in the 1970s.[7] In one experiment, Simon tested a group of chess players: one expert player, one intermediate player and one novice. He showed them a series of chess boards taken from the middle of a real game for a brief period of about 2–10 seconds, and then asked them to reproduce the 25 pieces on the board from memory. The expert chess player was able to reproduce two-thirds of the pieces correctly, on average. The intermediate player recalled fewer than half the pieces, while the novice could only recall about 5 pieces accurately, on average. At first glance, this seems to suggest something about the superior memory of chess experts. However, Simon went on to repeat the experiment but with one crucial difference. This time, he used the same number of chess pieces, but he placed them at random on the board rather than copying positions from an actual game. In this experiment, the novices and the experts all performed equally poorly and were only able to remember two or three pieces on average. The implication of this famous and significant experiment is that skill is not easily transferred, even to very similar domains. The ability of the chess experts to memorise a board of pieces and to reason their way through a chess problem is not a generic skill that can transfer to other problems, even when those problems are very similar. And that is not just true of chess, as E.D. Hirsch makes clear in his commentary on this research:

> *This experiment has been duplicated in several different laboratories, and structurally in several other fields, including algebra, physics and medicine, always with the same striking results. When the configuration of a task is significantly changed, past skills are not transferred to the new problem. In normal circumstances, of course, elements from past problems appear in present ones, and experts perform well with duplicated elements. But beyond similar or analogous circumstances, skill is not transferred.*
>
> Hirsch Jr., E.D., *Cultural Literacy: What Every American Needs to Know*, p.61

One of the reasons why skill does not transfer in this way is because it is domain-specific. Complex skills depend on very specific mental models, not generic ones which can be applied to very different areas. For example, Simon built on the results of his experiments on chess players to suggest that expert chess players have between 10,000 and 100,000 chunks of chess positions stored in long-term memory.[7] That is where a grandmaster's chess expertise derives from, not from an abstract reasoning muscle. In other fields of expertise, something similar is true: research in fields as varied as physics, electronics, reading, bridge-playing, typing and computer programming demonstrate the same principle.[8] Experts in every field depend on rich and detailed structures of knowledge stored in their long-term memory. These structures – often called schema or mental models – are what allow the expert to encounter new problems and solve them with such ease.

The reason why these mental models in long-term memory are so important is because long-term memory is one of the most powerful parts of human cognitive architecture, capable of storing vast quantities of information.[9] When we want to think or solve problems, we can call on resources from long-term memory, and also from working memory. Working memory, which can be equated with consciousness, is where we hold all the things we are thinking about at a particular moment in time. Unfortunately, it is highly limited. There is some debate in the literature about exactly how limited it is, but some of the most recent research suggests that it may be limited to as few as three or four items.[10–12] This means that relying solely on working memory to solve problems is not very effective. We need the help provided by the mental models stored in long-term memory and in order to get that help we need to acquire such mental models in the first place.

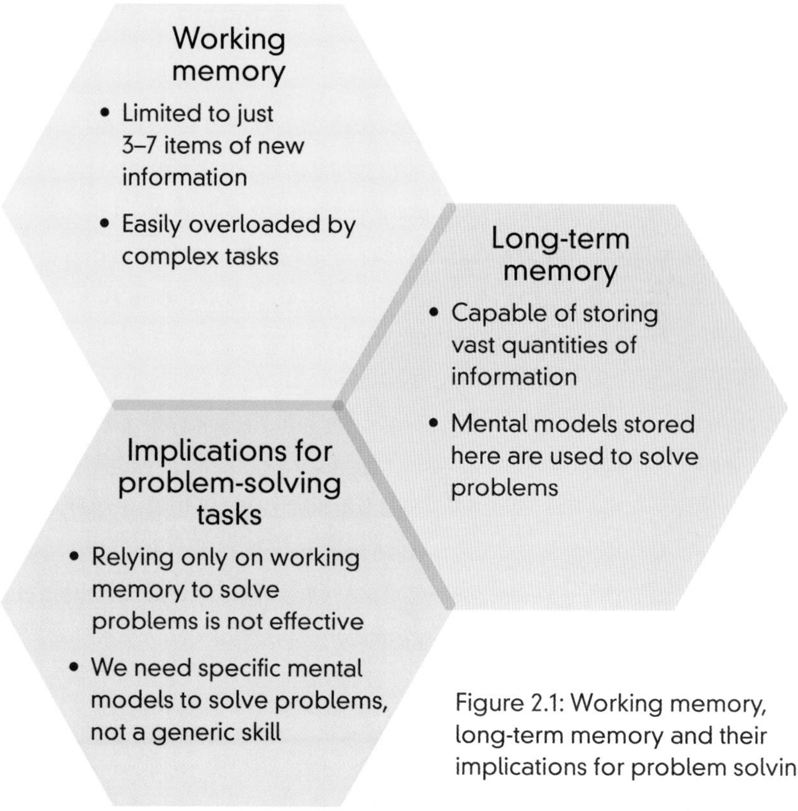

Working memory
- Limited to just 3–7 items of new information
- Easily overloaded by complex tasks

Long-term memory
- Capable of storing vast quantities of information
- Mental models stored here are used to solve problems

Implications for problem-solving tasks
- Relying only on working memory to solve problems is not effective
- We need specific mental models to solve problems, not a generic skill

Figure 2.1: Working memory, long-term memory and their implications for problem solving

We will look at how we acquire such mental models later in this chapter. For now, the important thing to note is that these mental models are specific, not generic.

The research against generic, transferable skills can feel quite counter-intuitive. This is perhaps particularly the case when it comes to science. After all, isn't one of the most important inventions of science the scientific method? And isn't one of the most important parts of that scientific method a set of habits of thinking, or skills, that can be applied to all content? Isn't it therefore legitimate to organise lessons around getting pupils to think and behave like scientists rather than around the scientific content itself? This reasoning is probably why 'thinking like a scientist' is perhaps one of the most popular transferable skills. But as Professor Daniel Willingham, a cognitive scientist, shows, even thinking like a scientist depends on knowledge of the specific scientific topic in question:

> For example, consider devising a research hypothesis. One could generate multiple hypotheses for any given situation. Suppose you know that car A gets better gas mileage than car B and you'd like to know why. There are many differences between the cars, so which will you investigate first? Engine size? Tire pressure? A key determinant of the hypothesis you select is plausibility. You won't choose to investigate a difference between cars A and B that you think is unlikely to contribute to gas mileage (e.g. paint color), but if someone provides a reason to make this factor more plausible (e.g. the way your teenage son's driving habits changed after he painted his car red), you are more likely to say that this now-plausible factor should be investigated. One's judgment about the plausibility of a factor being important is based on one's knowledge of the domain.
>
> Willingham, D.T., *Critical Thinking*, p.16

Another way of looking at this is that, when devising a hypothesis and interpreting data, recognising and interpreting anomalies is absolutely central, and recognising and interpreting anomalies depends, by definition, on knowing what is not an anomaly. Even reading, which seems to be the archetypal transferable skill, is more domain-specific than we might think at first. Many research studies have shown that, when we read, we are dependent on knowledge of vocabulary and of background knowledge about the topic in question.[13–18] Even good readers of English can be stymied if they come across an article with an unfamiliar context or vocabulary, such as a photocopier manual, or a newspaper column discussing an unfamiliar sport.

The implication of this research for education, and for the effectiveness of the kinds of lessons described at the start of this chapter, is profound. Those lessons had a cross-curricular focus on competencies such as managing information or forming hypotheses. They were based on the theory that there is such a thing as a generic, transferable skill. This incorrect theory leads to a practical flaw: it means that such lessons are too careless about the exact content that is included in them. If there is no such thing as a transferable skill, then suddenly the specifics of the content that is taught start to become very important again. Teaching pupils how to manage information in the context of some work on map skills does not guarantee that they will be able to manage information in the context of a nineteenth-century novel, or vice versa. The insight from cognitive psychology is that the specifics matter. If we care about pupils being able to manage information from map skills and nineteenth-century novels, then we will need to teach it. Pupils can't learn to think like scientists in any meaningful sense unless they actually engage with scientific content. Pupils can't become successful readers without the vocabulary and background knowledge that is commonly referred to in most texts. However, in many cases, as we saw, these lessons were deliberately unconcerned about the specifics of the content because they focused so much on the apparently transferable skill.

Similarly, the suggestion in one of the Ofsted lessons that a pupil might be able to 'assess their development against defined competencies, weekly or in individual lessons' across different projects is also called into question by this research.[19] As we've seen, when the content changes significantly, skill does not transfer. So the idea that one can build up skill across very different content and expect to see a smooth, linear progression is also flawed. This is even the case if one is trying to track the development of a skill within a subject. A pupil may be excellent at analysing non-fiction texts, but much less good at analysing a Shakespearean text simply because they have more familiarity and knowledge of the kind of vocabulary and context referred to in non-fiction texts. To get better at their analysis of Shakespearean texts, they don't need to improve their generic skills of analysis but to improve their knowledge and understanding of Shakespearean texts.

Of course, in everyday life, we do talk of our pupils, and indeed adults, as being good readers, or good problem solvers, or good critical thinkers. The people who we describe in this way are generally those with a wide background knowledge such that they are able to make sense of a wide range of different problems that come their way. The same is true in other areas. To the extent that professional historians are able to analyse a source that is not from their field of expertise, what matters is not their generic ability to do historical analysis, but their knowledge of the particular era in question. It is therefore still a legitimate aim of schooling to try and develop skills such as literacy, numeracy, problem solving and critical thinking. It is just that we need to accept that in doing so, we have to pay a lot more attention to the specific domains we want pupils to be skilled in, as well as to the specific areas of content we will have to teach in order for them to achieve this. In this sense, as Herbert Simon has noted, the language we use to describe highly skilled individuals is often misleading, in that it makes it sound as though expertise derives from generic skill, not from specific mental models.[20]

We can see that one significant problem with this generic-skill approach is that it suggests skills are transferable and, as a result, it is careless about the type of knowledge that is to be taught. However, advocates of these kinds of project-based lessons might argue that this problem is not a fundamental one. After all, they might say, it is perfectly possible to learn specific knowledge through such projects. Surely it would be possible to structure such projects so that pupils were getting all the important knowledge they needed through such tasks?

As long as sufficient care is given to the structure and type of knowledge presented in the project, the project-based approach can still work. This might particularly be the case when we consider that the same research which discusses the importance of mental models also talks about the importance of practice. Acquiring these mental models is not a passive but an active process. In order for knowledge to 'stick' in long-term memory, pupils have to make such knowledge their own and incorporate it into their mental models. Given that this is the case, is the best method of acquiring such mental models to do some of the activities outlined at the start of this chapter, such as creating a radio soap opera? In the next part of this chapter, we'll consider the type of practice that best helps to develop the mental models necessary for skill.

Practice needs to be deliberate

It is true that these kinds of project-based, generic-skill lessons allow pupils the chance to practise. And it is also true that practice is absolutely vital for skill development. However, this brings us on to the second reason why the generic-skill method is flawed. Practice is vital for skill development, but not all practice is equally important or effective. The type of practice that is most effective at developing skill is very specific and focused; it does not involve the broader and more complex activities recommended by the generic-skill model.

The foremost researcher on practice is K. Anders Ericsson, Professor of Psychology at Florida State University. He has shown that the best way to develop skill is through what he terms 'deliberate practice': a highly structured activity, the explicit goal of which is to improve performance. Specific tasks are invented to overcome weaknesses, and performance is carefully monitored to provide cues for ways to improve it further.[21] Ericsson draws a distinction between work, or performance, and deliberate practice. Work activities offer some opportunities for learning, but these opportunities are constrained because of the focus on performance. Deliberate practice, on the other hand, is designed with learning in mind. The following example shows the differences between the two:

> *Let us briefly illustrate the differences between work and deliberate practice. During a 3-hr baseball game, a batter may get only 5-15 pitches (perhaps one or two relevant to a particular weakness), whereas during optimal practice of the same duration, a batter working with a dedicated pitcher has several hundred batting opportunities, where this weakness can be systematically explored.*
>
> Ericsson, K.A., Krampe, R.T. and Tesch-Römer, C.: *'The role of deliberate practice in the acquisition of expert performance'.* Psychological Review 1993; 100: p.368

Ericsson has shown that this distinction between deliberate practice and performance holds across a number of fields. Skill is developed not by practising performances or final tasks, but by practising much narrower and more specific tasks. Baseball players do not practise batting by playing games over and over and over again. Concert musicians do not practise by doing and redoing performance pieces. Footballers don't practise by playing 11-a-side games, but by doing passing drills and small-sided games which are different to the final performance. Chess players don't practise by playing entire games, but by studying decomposed problems, and textbook openings and endings.

The aim of this deliberate practice is to build up the mental models discussed earlier. Narrow and focused practice is more effective at developing these mental models than broader and more complex practice. The reason for this is also related to the limitations of working memory. As we've seen, our working memories are limited, and the only way we can expand them is to draw on the resources we have in long-term memory. Novices, who lack such resources, are entirely reliant on limited working memory. So, when novices are asked to carry out complex problems or performances, the effort frequently overloads working memory.

By contrast, deliberate practice respects the limits of working memory and allows the learner to direct all of their attention on one specific aspect of performance. This kind of focus is also what enables feedback to be most effective. Compare the feedback that baseball players could receive in Ericsson's example with the feedback they might receive in a game situation. In the deliberate-practice example, baseball batters can ask for a series of pitches that target a particular weakness. They can receive immediate feedback from the pitcher as well as from their own observation and then they can react to that feedback immediately, too. In a game situation, the baseball batter will receive a variety of different pitches. The batter may or may not self-diagnose a particular weakness when facing a particular type of pitch and will almost certainly not have the opportunity to act on that feedback in the game situation. Game situations do not offer the potential for diagnosis or improvement that practice situations do, because they place such a burden on working memory.

This means that, even if pupils do manage to struggle through a difficult problem and perform well on it, there is a good chance that they will not have learnt much from the experience. This is because, ultimately, the mental activities required to solve a problem do not always help with the construction of mental models:

Solving a problem requires problem-solving search and search must occur using our limited working memory. Problem-solving search is an inefficient way of altering long-term memory because its function is to find a problem solution, not alter long-term memory. Indeed, problem-solving search can function perfectly with no learning whatsoever (Sweller, 1988). Thus, problem-solving search overburdens limited working memory and requires working memory resources to be used for activities that are unrelated to learning. As a consequence, learners can engage in problem-solving activities for extended periods and learn almost nothing (Sweller et al., 1982).

Kirschner, P. A., Sweller, J. and Clark, R.E.,
Why Minimal Guidance During Instruction Does Not Work, p.80

This also shows us that it is possible for a pupil to be thinking hard and struggling but still not learning. The reverse is also true: it is possible for a pupil to find something relatively straightforward but still to be learning. Professor Robert Bjork and other researchers have found that even if a pupil's performance on a particular task is perfect, it can still be worthwhile for them to continue to learn or practise something.[22] This 'overlearning' is valuable because it helps to strengthen and consolidate the mental models in long-term memory. However, it can often be hard to detect if we only look at performance on a task. In Bjork's words: '...that performance is often fleeting and, consequently, a highly imperfect index of learning does not appear to be appreciated by learners or instructors who frequently misinterpret short-term performance as a guide to long-term learning.'[22]

In order to distinguish between the types of tasks that do cause learning and the types that don't, we need to be clear about exactly what learning is and how it is different from performance. Learning can be defined as a change in long-term memory, and the aims of learning and the aims of performance are different.[23] Performance depends on the detailed, knowledge-rich mental models stored in long-term memory.

The aim of performance is to use those mental models. The aim of learning is to create them. The activities which create such models often don't look like the performance itself. In the words of Kirschner, Sweller and Clark, 'the practice of a profession is not the same as learning to practice the profession.'[23]

Again, the implications of this for the generic-skill method of instruction are significant. As we've seen, the generic-skill method is based on the idea that practising the final, complex, authentic skill will help pupils get better. Take, for example, the lesson that Ofsted praised because it featured a realistic writers' meeting:

> *The meeting was a remarkably successful and realistic one, taking on*
> *all the elements of the kind of writers' meeting that you might get as*
> *part of a real TV or radio soap opera.*
>
> Ofsted, *Moving English forward: Action to raise standards in English,* pp.52–53

If we consider this in the light of the research referenced earlier, its realism becomes not a point in its favour, but a point against it. Copying what experts do is not actually a good way of becoming an expert. Lessons which require students to think like a scientist or mathematician will not actually equip pupils with the mental models they need to actually think like a scientist or mathematician. The dominant generic-skill model of instruction is based on the flawed premise that practising the final skill will improve the final skill. In actual fact, not only are such activities not the best way of developing the final skill, but in many cases they are actually counter-productive.

Paradoxically, methods of teaching which ask pupils to do real and complex tasks will prevent pupils from developing the mental models they need to actually be able to solve those real and complex tasks. Pupils will be caught in a chicken-and-egg scenario: unable to solve complex problems because they do not have the necessary models, but unable to develop those models because they spend all of their time attempting to solve complex problems.

Indeed, in a paper from 1980, Simon noted this kind of circular reasoning that confused the description of a phenomenon with its explanation:

> *The magic of words is such that, when we are unable to explain*
> *a phenomenon, we sometimes find a name for it, as Molière's*
> *physician 'explained' the effects of opium by its dormitive property.*
> *So we 'explain' superior problem-solving skill by calling it 'talent',*
> *'intuition', 'judgment' and 'imagination'.*
>
> Larkin, J., McDermott, J., Simon, D.P. and Simon, H.A.,
> *Expert and novice performance in solving physics problems*, p.1335

It is exactly this kind of circular reasoning that leads us to hope that telling pupils to 'look at an issue from both sides' or 'look for countervailing evidence' will lead to them actually being able to do so. As Willingham notes, 'if you remind a student to "look at an issue from multiple perspectives" often enough, he will learn that he ought to do so, but if he doesn't know much about an issue, he can't think about it from multiple perspectives.'[24] And it is this same circular reasoning that leads to the problem noted by Wiliam in the previous chapter: the problem of teachers giving feedback that is accurate but not helpful, descriptive but not analytic, summative but not formative. Feedback such as "You need to be more systematic in planning your scientific inquiries" is just as unhelpful as being told that you need to look at an issue from multiple perspectives.[25] However, as long as we subscribe to the generic-skill model of instruction, then such feedback will be all that is possible. Only when we accept it is possible for complex skills to be broken down into smaller chunks will more precise, specific, and therefore helpful, feedback be possible.

An alternative method: deliberate practice

If the generic-skill method does not actually help to develop skill, what method would help? In the context of sport, Wiliam suggests the following:

> *The coach has to design a series of activities that will move athletes from their current state to the goal state. Often coaches will take a complex activity, such as the double play in baseball, and break it down into a series of components, each of which needs to be practiced until fluency is reached, and then the components are assembled together. Not only does the coach have a clear notion of quality (the well-executed double play), he also understands the anatomy of quality; he is able to see the high-quality performance as being composed of a series of elements that can be broken down into a developmental sequence for the athlete. This skill of being able to break down a long learning journey—from where the student is right now to where she needs to be—into a series of small steps takes years for even the most capable coaches to develop.*
>
> Wiliam, D., *Embedded formative assessment,* p.120

Wiliam goes on to describe this process as creating a 'model of progression'. How would this work in education? What do 'models of progression' look like in common school subjects? There are a number of educational approaches which take into account much of the research presented earlier and which consequently have had a great deal of success. Perhaps one of the most successful approaches is 'direct instruction', described by the educationalist John Hattie as follows:

> *In a nutshell: The teacher decides the learning intentions and success criteria, makes them transparent to the students, demonstrates them by modelling, evaluates if they understand what they have been told by checking for understanding, and re-telling them what they have told by tying it all together with closure.*
>
> Hattie, J., *Visible learning,* p.206

Some specific direct instruction programmes have been developed by Siegfried Engelmann, an American educationalist. One of them, Expressive Writing, offers an interesting contrast to the kinds of English lessons that we saw were praised by Ofsted. Whereas those lessons generally tended to involve pupils doing lots of writing, Expressive Writing breaks down the skill of writing into a number of quite small and specific tasks, and then gets pupils to practise those over and over again in different contexts.[26]

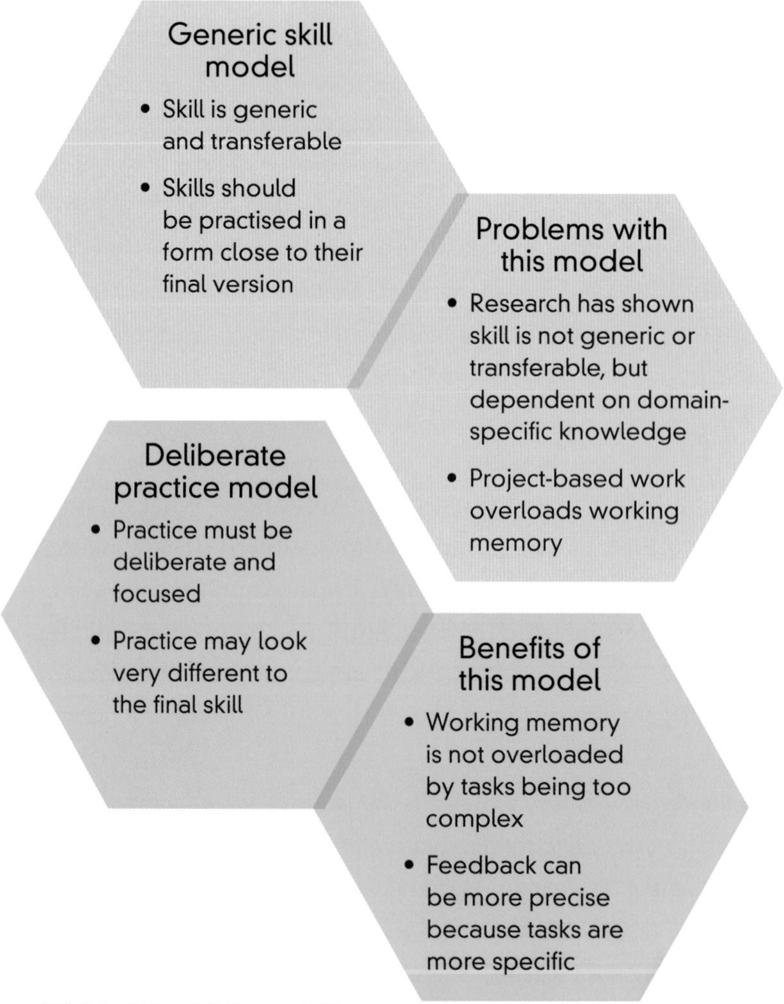

Generic skill model

- Skill is generic and transferable
- Skills should be practised in a form close to their final version

Problems with this model

- Research has shown skill is not generic or transferable, but dependent on domain-specific knowledge
- Project-based work overloads working memory

Deliberate practice model

- Practice must be deliberate and focused
- Practice may look very different to the final skill

Benefits of this model

- Working memory is not overloaded by tasks being too complex
- Feedback can be more precise because tasks are more specific

Figure 2.2: Models of skill acquisition

It has a specific and clearly detailed model of progression, similar to that of the baseball coach Wiliam refers to. For example, the very early activities require pupils to replace a present-tense verb with one in the past tense. There are many activities on rewriting sentences so that the use of pronouns is consistent and unambiguous. There are others on avoiding run-on sentences. At the end of each lesson, there is a structured writing activity which asks pupils to apply the lessons they have learnt earlier on. The way that the final skill is decomposed into small constituent parts is consistent with the deliberate-practice approach outlined earlier. There is substantial evidence to show that Engelmann's programmes, and direct-instruction approaches more generally, are much more effective than the generic-skill approaches outlined at the start of the chapter.

Using pupil self- and peer-assessment

These direct instruction programmes also include lots of opportunities for pupils to assess their own work and to share it with other pupils in the class. This is also vital because we've seen that formative assessment is not just about teachers responding to information about pupil progress, but it is also about pupils being responsive and becoming owners of their own learning. However, self-assessing and peer-assessing complex tasks is not straightforward.

Psychological studies show that those who lack competence in a particular domain also lack the ability to make judgements about their own performance. In a series of experiments on college students, the psychologists David Dunning and Justin Kruger showed that students who did poorly on tests of logical reasoning and English grammar also did poorly when asked to rate their own ability in such areas.[27] They persistently overestimated the number of questions they got right on such tests. Fascinatingly, their poor judgement about their own ability persisted even after they were given the completed test papers of stronger students to review. The only thing that did help them to improve was instruction in the domain itself.

This experiment, and others like it, has huge implications for our use of peer- and self-assessment in the classroom. First, it reinforces the importance of self- and peer-assessment and of metacognition. Being able to tell the difference between competence and incompetence is actually an aspect of developing competence. Developing our pupils' ability involves developing their ability to perceive quality. Second, it suggests that we have to design peer- and self-assessment tasks that are within the level of competence of our pupils. That is to say, we cannot expect them to peer- and self-assess complex tasks. Third, it suggests that we need to think carefully about how we use examples of excellent work. We cannot assume that simply being shown excellent work is enough to develop excellence. Something more is needed: either the complex task needs to be broken down, or particular aspects of a quality piece of work need to be explicitly highlighted and emphasised by a teacher. Direct instruction programmes use self-assessment and peer-assessment in these more sophisticated ways.

In conclusion, the research about skill development shows us that in order to develop skill, we need lots of specific knowledge and lots of deliberate practice at using that knowledge. There is no catch-all, all-purpose generic ability we can acquire. Specific detail is what matters. It is perhaps for this reason that direct instruction has been described as being about 'attention to picky, picky detail.'[28] Attention to such 'picky, picky detail' can feel pedantic – and even irrelevant – but it is crucial. When we are novices, it is hard for us to appreciate the exact importance of such detail, which is why we need a lot of guidance and direction.

Memorising and practising the right things

Throughout this chapter, we've looked at the value of knowledge in developing skill. One common criticism of the way knowledge is taught in education is that it is possible for pupils to know something and yet not to do it. For example, most pupils at secondary school know that they should begin a sentence with a capital letter and, if you ask them how to start a sentence, most of them will give you the correct answer. However, many fewer pupils do consistently start a sentence with a capital letter. For many, therefore, this is a good example of why traditional teaching methods based on knowledge transmission are not effective. Pupils *know* things, but they don't *do* them. We might term this problem, and other similar ones, a 'knowing-doing gap'.[29] Pupils – and indeed, in many cases, adults – know what they are supposed to do, yet they don't do it reliably.

Research shows that this knowing-doing gap is widespread, and not just in education.[30] The important question then becomes: how does one close the gap? The response of the generic-skill model is to say that if pupils do enough real-world tasks and are introduced to enough real-world models, they will pick up the correct way of doing things. However, there is no evidence that this will close the knowing-doing gap because, as we've seen, these real-world tasks overwhelm working memory. There are so many things to learn from these experiences that it is impossible to take them all in at once.

The method that has more success in closing this knowing-doing gap is the deliberate-practice method. This method is based around the isolation and practice of the particular subskill one wants pupils to be able to do. In the case of the capital letter, the best approach would be to set up a series of activities that require pupils to use the capital letter correctly. For example, pupils might write out four or five simple sentences that use capitals correctly. Then they might be asked to read ten sentences and identify and correct the five that use capitals incorrectly. Next, they might be asked to write a short paragraph based on a series of pictures, and to focus specifically on using capitals correctly. Such a series of lessons are a long way from lessons where pupils repeat 'sentences begin with a capital letter' over and over again. But such lessons are also a long way from the popular and dominant generic-skill lessons recommended by so many in English education.

Another way of conceptualising the knowing-doing gap question might be that it is less a gap between knowing and doing, and more a question of isolating, memorising and practising the right kind of knowledge. Indeed, in Engelmann's terms, it is about attention to the 'picky, picky detail'. Memorising the rule book is rarely the best way to master any kind of skill, just as we shall see later that memorising rubrics is rarely the best way to understand what quality is. But just because memorising rule books is not optimal for developing skill, it does not mean that all knowledge and memorisation is therefore redundant. Nor does it mean that we can rely on real-world contexts to learn everything we need. Another good example of this can be seen by comparing different methods of learning vocabulary. The best way to learn vocabulary is not to read or to memorise dictionary definitions. However, we still do need to commit vocabulary to memory. It is just that it is better to learn vocabulary through carefully constructed sentence examples, rather than through dictionary definitions.[31]

Implications for assessment

To sum up, in this chapter we've looked at the dominant generic-skill approach to teaching skill. We've seen that research from cognitive science shows that such an approach is flawed because it assumes that skills are transferable and that the best kind of practice is of complex performances. We've seen instead that the deliberate-practice model is more effective. The deliberate-practice model focusses on building the specific knowledge and mental models required for high-level skill, and, in doing so, focuses practice on tasks and activities that do not look like the final skill.

We can see already that these two different methods of teaching have significant implications for AfL. As we've seen in Chapter 1, AfL is about the process and method of learning, not the outcome. So different ideas about the process and method of learning will lead to fundamentally different conceptions of AfL. In short, the deliberate-practice model suggests we need to use different tasks depending on whether we are assessing for formative or summative purposes, whereas the generic-skill model suggests that the same task can fulfil both purposes. In the next chapter, we will consider this issue in more depth but from the point of view of assessment theory.

Notes

1 Claxton, G., 2006. *Expanding the Capacity to Learn: A new end for education?* British Educational Research Association Annual Conference, 6 September, Warwick University, p.2, <https://www.decd.sa.gov.au/sites/g/files/net691/f/expanding_the_capacity_to_learn_a_new_end_for_education.pdf> accessed 19 August 2016

2 RSA Opening Minds. <https://www.thersa.org/action-and-research/rsa-projects/creative-learning-and-development-folder/opening-minds> accessed 19 August 2016

3 RSA Opening Minds, 2002. *RSA Opening Minds Project Handbook.* London: RSA, p.4 <http://www.creativetallis.com/uploads/2/2/8/7/2287089/opening_minds_handbook.pdf> accessed 19 August 2016

4 Boyle, H., 2006. *Opening Minds: A competency-based curriculum for the twenty first century. National Teacher Research Panel,* p.3 <www.ntrp.org.uk/sites/all/documents/HBSummary.pdf> accessed 19 August 2016

5 Christodoulou, D., 2014. *Seven Myths about Education.* London: Routledge. Lesson descriptions are taken from the following Ofsted subject reports: *Making a mark: art, craft and design education 2008–11,* March 2012; *Moving English forward: Action to raise standards in English,* March 2012; *Excellence in English: What we can learn from 12 outstanding schools,* May 2011; *Geography: Learning to make a world of difference,* February 2011; *History for all: History in English schools 2007/10,* March 2011; *Mathematics: Made to measure,* May 2012; *Modern languages: Achievement and challenge 2007–2010,* January 2011; *Transforming religious education: Religious education in schools 2006–09,* June 2010; *Successful science: An evaluation of science education in England 2007–2010,* January 2011

6 de Groot, A.D., 1978. *Thought and Choice in Chess.* The Hague: Mouton

7 Simon, H. and Chase, W., 1973. Skill in chess. *American Scientist,* 61, pp.394–403

8 Feltovich, P.J., Prietula, M.J. and Ericsson, K.A., 2006. Studies of Expertise from Psychological Perspectives. In Ericsson, K.A et al., eds. *The Cambridge Handbook of Expertise and Expert Performance.* Cambridge: Cambridge University Press, pp.41–67

9 Sweller, J., van Merriënboer, J.J.G. and Paas, F.G.W.C., 1998. Cognitive Architecture and Instructional Design. *Educational Psychology Review,* 10, pp.251–296

10 Cowan, N, 2001. The magical number 4 in short-term memory: A reconsideration of mental storage capacity. *Behavioral and Brain Sciences,* 24, pp.87–114

11 Cowan, N., 2005. *Working Memory Capacity: Essays in Cognitive Psychology.* Hove: Taylor and Francis

12 See also Miller, G.A, 1956. The Magical Number Seven, Plus or Minus Two: Some Limits on Our Capacity for Processing Information. *Psychological Review,* 63, pp.81–97

13 Recht, D.R and Leslie, L, 1988. Effect of prior knowledge on good and poor readers' memory of text. *Journal of Educational Psychology,* 80, pp.16–20

14 Pearson, P.D., 1979. The Effect of Background Knowledge on Young Children's

Comprehension of Explicit and Implicit Information. *Journal of Literacy Research*, 11, pp.201–209

15 Taft, M.L and Leslie, L., 1985. The Effects of Prior Knowledge and Oral Reading Accuracy on Miscues and Comprehension. *Journal of Reading Behavior*, 17, pp.163–179

16 Taylor, B.M., 1979. Good and Poor Readers' Recall of Familiar and Unfamiliar Text. *Journal of Literacy Research*, 11, pp.375–380

17 McNamara, D. and Kintsch, W., 1996. Learning from texts: Effect of prior knowledge and text coherence. *Discourse Processes*, 22, pp.247–288

18 Caillies, S., Denhière, G. and Kintsch, W., 2002. The Effect of prior knowledge on understanding from text: Evidence from primed recognition. *European Journal of Cognitive Psychology*, 14, pp.267–286

19 Ofsted, 2008. *Curriculum innovation in schools,* pp.9–10 <http://www.readyunlimited.com/wp-content/uploads/2015/09/Curriculum-Innovation-in-schools-ofsted.pdf> accessed 19 August 2016

20 Larkin, J., McDermott, J., Simon, D.P. and Simon, H.A, 1980. Expert and Novice Performance in Solving Physics Problems. *Science*, 208(4450), pp.1335–1342

21 Ericsson, K.A, Krampe, R.T. and Tesch-Römer, C., 1993. The Role of Deliberate Practice in the Acquisition of Expert Performance, *Psychological Review*, 100, pp.363–406

22 Soderstrom, N.C. and Bjork, R.A, 2013. Learning versus performance. In Dunn, D.S., ed. *Oxford bibliographies online: Psychology.* New York: Oxford University Press

23 Kirschner, P.A, Sweller, J. and Clark, R.E., 2006. Why Minimal Guidance During Instruction Does Not Work: An Analysis of the Failure of Constructivist, Discovery, Problem-Based, Experiential, and Inquiry-Based Teaching. *Educational Psychologist*, 41, pp.75–86

24 Willingham, D.T., 2007. Critical thinking. *American Educator*, Summer 2007

25 Wiliam, D., 2011. *Embedded formative assessment.* Indiana: Solution Tree Press, p.120

26 Engelmann, S. and Silbert, J., 2005. *Expressive Writing 1.* Ohio: SRA/McGraw-Hill

27 Kruger, J. and Dunning, D., 1999. Unskilled and Unaware of It: How Difficulties in Recognizing One's Own Incompetence Lead to Inflated Self-Assessments. *Journal of Personality and Social Psychology*, 77(6), p.1121

28 Quoted in Ashman, G., 2016. A day at researchED Melbourne. *Filling the pail*, 22 May [Blog] <https://gregashman.wordpress.com/2016/05/22/a-day-at-researched-melbourne/> accessed 19 August 2016

29 Jeffrey Pfeffer and Robert Sutton use this phrase as the title of their book on management, *The Knowing-Doing Gap: How Smart Companies Turn Knowledge into Action.* Wellesley, Massachusetts: Harvard Business Press, 2013

30 See Pfeffer and Sutton, op. cit., and Ericsson, A and Pool, R, 2016. *Peak: Secrets from the New Science of Expertise.* London: Bodley Head, Chapter 5

31 Miller, G.A and Gildea, P.M., 1987. How children learn words. *Scientific American*, 257, pp.94–99

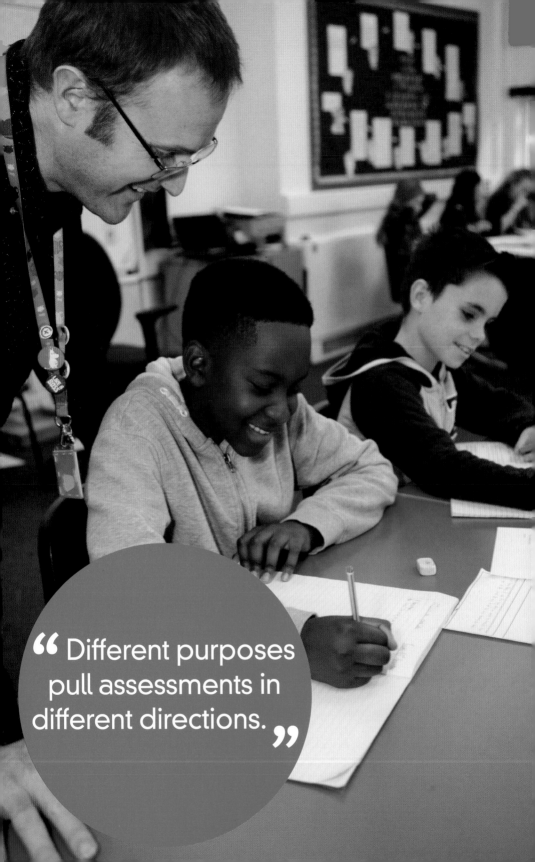

"Different purposes pull assessments in different directions."

Making valid inferences

3

Meanings and consequences

In the last two chapters, we looked at evidence from cognitive psychology which showed that the best way to develop skill is to break it down into small pieces. As a result, it is hard to rely on the same task, or even the same type of task, for both formative and summative purposes. In this chapter, we will look at what assessment theory has to say about a similar question: to what extent can the same task be used to provide formative and summative information?

Interestingly, Wiliam and Black considered this same question in a paper written not long before *Inside the Black Box*. The title of the paper, 'Meanings and Consequences', refers to what they feel are the differences between the formative and summative purposes of assessments. For Wiliam and Black, the purpose of assessing summatively is to produce a shared meaning. The purpose of assessing formatively is to produce a consequence for the teacher and pupil.[1]

For example, when we assess summatively, we 'judge the extent of students' learning of the material in a course, for the purpose of grading, certification, evaluation of progress or even for researching the effectiveness of a curriculum.'[1] When making these summative judgements, it is vitally important that they have some kind of shared meaning that goes beyond the context in which they were made.

Such judgements have to be shared and consistent across different schools, different teachers and different pupils. We have to be confident that a pupil who is given a particular summative judgement in one school would have received a similar one in another school. In Wiliam and Black's words, 'summative functions prioritise the consistency of meanings across contexts and individuals.'[1] This is not easy, and we will go on to discuss the challenges involved in producing such shared meanings. The purpose of a formative assessment, by contrast, is to give teachers and pupils information that 'form[s] the basis for successful action in improving performance.'[1] That is, the purpose of a formative assessment is to provide useful consequences for teachers and pupils which give them a better idea about what they should do next.

In some ways it is possible to take an assessment that has been designed with one purpose in mind and to reuse it for another purpose. For example, 'the results of an assessment that had been designed originally to fulfil a summative function might be used formatively, as is the case when a teacher administers a paper from a previous year in order to help students to prepare for an examination.'[1] In this case, the evidence from the test can be used to produce a shared meaning, such as a grade, and some useful consequences, such as identifying certain areas of relative strength or weakness that a pupil needs to work on.

It is not always this simple. Different purposes pull assessments in different directions. An assessment may be perfectly designed for one purpose, but it may not work very well if it is asked to fulfil an entirely different one. For example, in a classroom discussion a pupil may display 'a frown of puzzlement' which leads the teacher to 'amend his or her approach almost instantaneously.'[1] In this case, the frown of puzzlement tells the teachers something extremely useful and allows them to adjust their teaching accordingly. That is, it provides useful consequences. However, a frown of puzzlement is of much less value in providing a shared summative meaning. The reverse is also true. Knowing that a pupil got a grade 'A' on a formal test is an accurate shared meaning, but it provides a teacher with relatively little information that will change their teaching.

For Wiliam and Black, therefore, this is not a binary issue, but a continuum. At the extremes there are some assessments which are simply not capable of fulfilling both formative and summative functions:

> *It would be very difficult to argue that responses to an 'off-the-cuff' question to a class in the middle of an episode of teaching would have any significance beyond the immediate context of the classroom. Conversely, evidence elicited at the end of a sequence of teaching can have very little formative influence on the students assessed.*
>
> Wiliam, D. and Black, P., *Meanings and Consequences*, p.546

In the middle of this continuum, there are some tasks which are capable of fulfilling more than one function, but Wiliam and Black are cautious about the identification of these tasks:

> *However, between these clear cases, it seems to us that there may be some common ground between the formative and summative functions. Finding this common ground will be difficult, since the issues are subtle and complex, and we have made only a small contribution here.*
>
> Wiliam, D. and Black, P., *Meanings and Consequences*, p.546

These issues are subtle and complex: the purpose to which an assessment is going to be put does impact on its design, which makes it harder to simplistically 'repurpose' assessments than it may first appear. And whilst it may be possible for some types of assessment to fulfil both functions, it may also be the case that this involves trade-offs; the assessment which is able to fulfil summative and formative purposes may not be ideal for either purpose. In order to evaluate the information we get from assessments, it is worth taking a detour at this point to explain two key assessment concepts: validity and reliability.

Validity

In the words of Daniel Koretz, Professor of Assessment at Harvard University, 'validity is the single most important criterion for evaluating achievement testing.'[2] Wiliam agrees, saying that it is 'the central concept in assessment'. He continues:

> *The really important idea here is that we are hardly ever interested in how well a student did on a particular assessment. What we are interested in is what we can say, from that evidence, about what the student can do in other situations, at other times, in other contexts. Some conclusions are warranted on the basis of the results of the assessment, and others are not. The process of establishing which kinds of conclusions are warranted and which are not is called validation.*
>
> Wiliam, D., *Principled Assessment Design*, p.22

For an example of this, think of a typical GCSE exam. In practice, most of the people who use the results of GCSE exams are not actually that interested in the exact questions a pupil got right or wrong in that particular test, at that particular time. If the only thing a GCSE exam could tell you is that between the hours of 1 p.m. and 3 p.m. on a day in June 2014, a pupil sat in an exam hall and answered 53% of maths questions correctly, it would not actually be that useful. What is useful is knowing that if a pupil did get that particular mark, at that particular time, we can be reasonably certain that they are, or are not, able to begin working at a job that requires basic numeracy or to start studying for a maths A level. These are the kinds of inferences we want to make from exams and, as Wiliam notes, we need to be sure that the exams we are using are capable of supporting such inferences. The process of doing this is called validation.

It is important to note, therefore, that validity refers not to a test or assessment itself, but to the inferences we make based on the test results.

> *Tests themselves are not valid or invalid. Rather, it is an inference based on test scores that is valid or not. A given test might provide good support for one inference, but weak support for another. For example, a well-designed end of course exam in statistics might provide good support for inferences about students' mastery of basic statistics, but very weak support for conclusions about mastery of mathematics more broadly.*
>
> Koretz, D., *Measuring Up*, p.31

In general, as both Wiliam and Koretz note, we are actually hardly ever interested in how well a pupil did on a particular assessment. We want to be able to make bigger and more significant inferences than this. Both the formative and summative inferences we discussed earlier involve trying to find out more than just how a pupil performed on one particular question, at one particular time.

Sampling

One difficult aspect concerning the validity of a test involves sampling. Summative inferences are typically about achievement in big subject areas, or domains. In a maths GCSE exam, for example, we are trying to make an inference about a pupil's ability in a huge domain. To assess everything a 16-year-old pupil knows about maths, we would need exams that were days, perhaps weeks, long, and the time and costs of such assessments would be prohibitive.[3] To get around this problem, examiners do not aim to test the entire domain. Instead, they aim to test a sample of the domain: 50 or 60 questions that can perhaps be answered in a couple of hours. Then, on the basis of a pupil's performance on those 50 or 60 questions, it is possible to make an inference about their wider maths ability.

Some assessments do not have to sample. In the early years, for example, we are sometimes interested in making summative inferences about domains that are so small they can be measured directly: letters of the alphabet or number bonds up to 10. However, as pupils grow older, generally the amount of content we are trying to measure increases, and most of the summative inferences we are interested in making are about domains that are so big that it is not possible to measure them directly. As a result, most assessments designed to produce a summative inference do not directly test the entire domain. So, when thinking about the validity of a summative inference we nearly always need to consider what the domain is we are trying to measure and how the test has sampled from that domain.

Reliability

One important aspect of validity is reliability. The marks and grades generated by assessments need to be reliable: that is, they need to 'show little inconsistency between one measurement and the next'.[2] When you weigh a kilogram bag of flour on a set of scales, if the scales are reliable, the scales should return a reading of 1 kilogram however many times you carry out the measurement. If they do, the scales are reliable. In educational measurement, a test is reliable if the scores are consistent.

For example:

- If a pupil were to take different versions of the same test, they should get approximately the same mark.
- If they were to take the test at different times of day, they should get approximately the same mark.

- If a pupil's answer paper were submitted to ten different markers, it should return each time with approximately the same mark.

These three instances should show how difficult it is for any exam to be perfectly reliable. They are three examples of the most common sources of unreliability.[4]

The first source is sampling unreliability. We can't keep reusing the same test because pupils will get used to it, so we have to create different versions that have different samples from the same domain. The sample of questions on one paper might, by chance, lead to a pupil doing a bit better or worse than they would have done on the sample on another paper. This is why, the night before an exam, so many of us hope that certain questions will and will not appear on the paper. We know that if we get a more favourable selection of questions on the exam paper we will end up doing better. This source of unreliability cannot be completely eliminated but it can be reduced by making the sample bigger, which often also means making the exam longer.

Another source of unreliability is student performance on the day. A pupil might do better or worse on an exam depending on when it is scheduled, how they are feeling, whether they have eaten breakfast or not, and dozens of other factors. This is a major factor in unreliability, and one that is perhaps the hardest to control.

A third source is marker unreliability. This type of unreliability varies depending on the types of questions included in the exam. Multiple-choice questions should have very low levels of marker unreliability: the same question should get the same mark, whoever marks it. However, exams which include lots of open tasks, like essays, tend to have higher levels of marker unreliability. It can be hard to ensure that different markers apply consistent standards, and even if they do, there may be legitimate disagreements between markers about the quality of an essay.

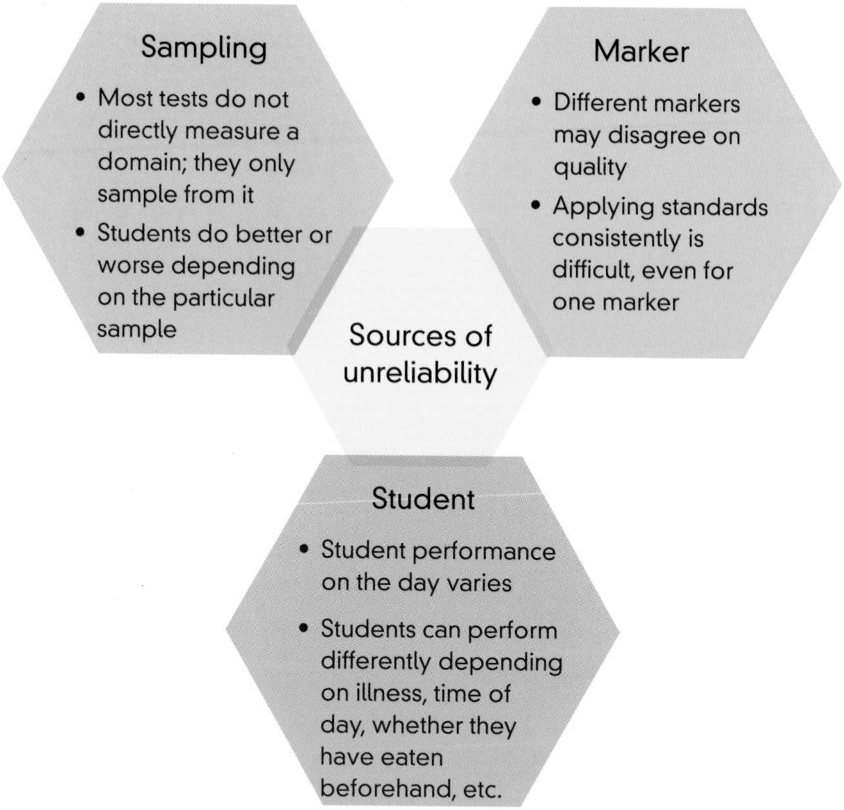

Sampling

- Most tests do not directly measure a domain; they only sample from it
- Students do better or worse depending on the particular sample

Marker

- Different markers may disagree on quality
- Applying standards consistently is difficult, even for one marker

Sources of unreliability

Student

- Student performance on the day varies
- Students can perform differently depending on illness, time of day, whether they have eaten beforehand, etc.

Figure 3.1: Sources of unreliability

We can see from this that it is impossible for any exam to be completely reliable. That is why some exams also give an idea of the range of scores that a pupil might have expected to achieve had they taken several sittings of the same exam. The anonymised report in Figure 3.2 from the New Group Reading Test (NGRT), shows this.[5] The NGRT is designed by GL Assessments, a UK provider of standardised educational assessments. The black dot represents the pupil's score on that particular test, but the horizontal black line shows the range of scores.

These sources of unreliability have important implications for measuring progress. On the report shown in Figure 3.2, Ben Arrosco

Student name	Age at test (yrs:mths)	SAS	SAS (90% confidence bands) 60 70 80 90 100 110 120 130 140	SAS difference	Progress category	S
Ben Arrosco	11:08	112		+2	Average	
	12:08	114				
Charlotte Benn-Agogo	11:07	128		+12	Above average	
	12:05	140				
Kate Beckett	11:06	115		+10	Above average	
	12:05	125				
Connor Callaghan	11:01	129		-2	Average	
	12:00	127				
Castle	11:05	104				

Figure 3.2: NGRT sample group progress report for teachers

scored 112 on the NGRT when he was 11, and then took a different version of the test a year later and got 114. On this kind of test, maintaining the same score over time represents average progress, and increasing a score represents above-average progress. However, although Ben has increased his score, it is by such a small amount that we cannot say with confidence that he has actually made above-average progress. His initial score of 112 was actually in the range of 102–118, and the follow-up score of 114 was in the range of 104–120. As a result, the report that comes with this test records his progress category as 'average'.

These three sources of unreliability affect different types of assessment in different ways. Two very common types of assessment are the quality model of assessment and the difficulty model. The quality model – often used in subjects like English language and literature, history, art, music and drama – requires the pupil to perform a task and then requires the marker to judge how well they have done it. Pupils might write an essay or a story, give a speech in a foreign language, or compose a piece of music. The difficulty model is more common in subjects like maths and science. It requires pupils to answer a series of different questions that increase in difficulty. Ayesha Ahmed and Alastair Pollitt, Research and Teaching Associate and Affiliate Lecturer at the University of Cambridge, give a sporting analogy which illustrates the difference between the two models:

To make the distinction between these two models clearer, consider two sporting paradigms that represent them well: ice dance (free skating) and high jump. Competitive ice dancing uses a pure quality model. All ice rinks are equally flat and roughly the same size, shape and temperature; in other words, the task is pretty much the same in every ice dance performance. The skater is expected to go out and perform in a way that impresses the judges as much as possible. In contrast, a high jump competition is a clear example of the difficulty model, consisting of a series of tasks of ever increasing difficulty which continues until everybody has failed. In the ice dance we focus on judging the responses, while in high jump we focus on counting successes on the tasks.

Ahmed, A. and Pollitt, A., *The Support Model for Interactive Assessment*, p.134

With the quality model, many of the problems with reliability come after the assessment has been completed: how sure can we be that all markers are applying consistent standards? In comparison, the difficulty model can seem more reliable because it is much easier to 'count success on the tasks'. However, it does also involve some tricky judgements. With this model, the difficult judgements involve the selection and creation of the questions themselves. In Ahmed and Pollitt's words:

The technical concern in the quality model is the reliability of the judges, whereas in the difficulty model it is the internal consistency of the questions. In assessing performance it is desirable that examiners are judging the same skills to the same standards, but achieving this is difficult and costly. In assessing understanding we need to know that every question is measuring the same trait or skills, and this also is very hard to guarantee.

Ahmed, A. and Pollitt, A., *The Support Model for Interactive Assessment*, p.134

In some ways, it could be argued that there is a trade-off between the reliability of an assessment and its validity. Sometimes, making

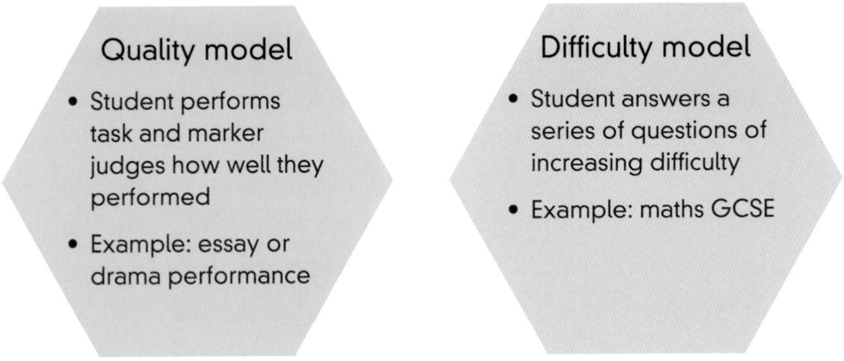

Quality model

- Student performs task and marker judges how well they performed
- Example: essay or drama performance

Difficulty model

- Student answers a series of questions of increasing difficulty
- Example: maths GCSE

Figure 3.3: The quality and difficulty models of assessment

an assessment more reliable reduces the validity of the inferences we want to be able to make. Writing is a good example: it is very hard to mark writing reliably. It is very easy, on the other hand, to mark a set of multiple-choice questions on grammar reliably. However, if we got rid of all writing assessments and replaced them with multiple-choice grammar questions we would be open to criticism that, by making the test more reliable, we had reduced the validity of the most common inferences people want to make from it. Most people who use the results of the test are not actually interested in the pupil's ability to answer multiple-choice questions about grammar. They want to know if the pupil can write. Changing the test may have made it more reliable, but it may no longer allow us to make the inference we are interested in.[6]

Whilst people often talk about the trade-off between reliability and validity, in actual fact the two are not at opposite ends of a spectrum. Whilst it is possible, as we have seen, to produce a highly reliable test that doesn't allow us to make valid inferences about the concepts we are interested in, the reverse is not true. It is not possible to produce a test which allows us to make valid inferences about the things we want which has low reliability. The lower the reliability of our test, the less valid are our inferences. For an example of this, let's look at writing again. Suppose, instead of assessing it through multiple-choice questions, we assessed it through a process of portfolio assessment, where pupils collect pieces of writing they have completed over a period of time in class and teachers mark the entire portfolio with a rubric. Such assessments seem as though they should be more valid, because they are closer to the kind of real-world abilities we are interested in. But they often produce very unreliable results: a pupil's mark may vary depending on the types of tasks they selected, the marker they are allocated, and the amount of help they have had with the task.[7] And because the results are not reliable, they cannot support any valid inferences either: what can we infer with confidence about a pupil with a certain grade if we are not certain they really deserve that grade?

It is all very well to create an exciting and open assessment task which corresponds to real-world tasks; however, if a pupil can end up with a wildly different mark depending on what task they are allocated, and who marks it, the mark cannot be used to support any valid inferences. Reliability is not some pettifogging and pedantic requirement: it is an aspect of validity, and a prerequisite for validity.[8] In the following discussion about making valid inferences, therefore, reliability will play an important part.

Valid summative and formative inferences

As we've seen, summative and formative inferences are quite different. A formative inference is one that provides useful and consequential information for teachers and pupils, whilst a summative inference provides a shared and consistent meaning across different contexts. Validating these different inferences, and in so doing, ensuring that they are reliable, also involves making different judgements.

Summative assessments are required to support large and broad inferences about how pupils will perform beyond the school and in comparison to their peers nationally. In order for such inferences to be valid, they need to be consistent – not just amongst a small group of pupils, but amongst pupils nationally – because they will be used by employers and universities to compare students from different schools and backgrounds.

The purpose of grades and other similar labelling systems is to provide an easy way of communicating this shared meaning. This is how GCSE grades work: in the old GCSE grading system, certain letters had shared meanings, and in the new GCSE grading system, numbers have shared meanings. A GCSE grade A* or grade 9 communicates a shared meaning about a pupil's ability in a subject. An employer or teacher at a further education college is able to infer from it how well the pupil has done in that subject. The old National Curriculum levels did the same. There are other methods of communicating a shared meaning which don't look like a grade but in practice fulfil the same function. For example, many new assessment systems have chosen to report performance in terms of labels such as 'emerging, expected and exceeding' or 'working in greater depth, working at the expected standard, and working below the expected standard'. In the report we looked at in Figure 3.2, from GL Assessment's NGRT, pupil scores are reported as a standard-age score, where 100 represents the average, and the scale runs from approximately 60 to 140.[9]

All these methods of reporting may look different, but they are all trying to communicate a shared meaning. Numbered grades, lettered grades, levels and standard age scores all have this in common. Shared meanings are not easy to create, and they impose restrictions on the design and administration of assessments. As Wiliam and Black say, when tests need to fulfil a summative function, 'shared meanings are much more important, and the considerable distortions and undesirable consequences that arise are often justified by appeal to the need to create consistency of interpretation.'[1] These distortions and undesirable consequences are significant, and it is worthwhile exploring some of them in more detail. In particular, in order to create a shared meaning, tests need to be taken in standard conditions, distinguish between pupils and measure large domains.

First, assessments which aim to produce shared meanings need to be taken in standard conditions with strict restrictions on the type of external help that is, and is not, available. This is to ensure that pupils in very different contexts and environments are treated consistently and fairly, and that their results are therefore comparable.[3]

Second, such assessments have to include questions that allow us to distinguish between different pupils. As Koretz says, 'discriminating items are simply needed if one wants to draw inferences about relative proficiency.'[3] This can be achieved in different ways, depending on the type of assessment. In the difficulty model of assessment, this involves including lots of questions of moderate difficulty. Koretz gives an example of a vocabulary test: one would not want to test the vocabulary of college students with words like 'bath', 'travel' or 'carpet'. All the students would get all the questions right, and this would tell you little about their relative proficiency. Neither would one want to test them with words like 'siliculose', 'vilipend' and 'epimysium'. All the students would get these wrong, and again, you would learn little about their relative proficiency. Instead, you want words like 'feckless', 'disparage' and 'minuscule'. As Koretz says, 'You want items of moderate difficulty that some of the students will answer correctly and some incorrectly.'[3] For the quality model of assessment, often used in English exams, pupils are asked to perform a complex task like writing an essay and the examiner judges how well they carry out the task. These two methods are different, but the aim is the same: to distinguish between all the candidates taking the assessment.

A third important restriction involves the amount of content an assessment has to cover. As Koretz argues, 'the tests that are of interest to policymakers, the press and the public…are designed to measure sizable domains, ranging from knowledge acquired over a year of study in a subject to cumulative mastery of material studied over several years.'[3] As we've seen, it isn't possible to measure such domains directly. Instead, assessments have to sample from that body of content: it will not be possible to cover all of it in a test that is a couple of hours long. Selecting the tasks that will form the sample, and ensuring that they are representative enough to allow for an inference about the domain, is a difficult task and one that imposes another restriction. These restrictions are significant but unfortunately unavoidable. All of these things are vital if the test is to provide a valid inference about how pupils are doing relative to their peers: that is, to provide a valid shared meaning.

As we've seen, the main inference that is needed from formative assessments is how we should proceed next. Validating this kind of inference is different. The assessment still needs to be reliable, because reliability is a prerequisite for validity. But these inferences do not need to be shared across different contexts, which makes achieving a high level of reliability much easier. I no longer need to be sure about how the pupils in my class match up to an external standard, or that the inference I am making would be shared by other teachers across the land. I just need to be sure that the inference I am making will help inform my next steps.

The restrictions outlined earlier do not apply. If I think it will give me useful information, I can give some pupils more help than others in answering a question; I certainly don't have to worry about whether I am giving them more or less help than pupils in a class next door, or in the next city. I don't have to worry about questions distinguishing between pupils: if I want to get useful information about what to do next, then a question everyone gets right or wrong might be very useful. Nor do I have to worry about questions or assessments covering an entire domain: a question which focuses on just one small part of a subject can be very helpful.

In general, therefore, it is possible to be much more flexible and responsive when designing assessments whose main purpose is formative. And being responsive is important: we saw in the first chapter that Wiliam wishes he had called formative assessment 'responsive teaching', because it involves adapting teaching based on feedback from pupils.[10] Often, these responses need to be made quickly, in the middle of a lesson. If teachers face the same restrictions when assessing formatively as examiners do when assessing summatively, it will not be possible for them to make these kinds of swift and responsive adjustments.

Examples

In order to illustrate these points, let's consider a couple of concrete examples of assessments which are good at providing one kind of inference, but not another. In his paper, 'Integrating formative and summative functions of assessment', Wiliam looks at the following maths example which shows a question that has flaws when used summatively but is useful when used formatively:

> *Simplify, if possible, 5a + 2b.*
> *Many teachers regard this as an unfair item, since students are*
> *'tricked' into simplifying the expression, because of the prevailing*
> *'didactic contract' (Brousseau, 1984) under which the students*
> *assume that there is 'academic work' (Doyle, 1983) to be done. In*
> *other words 'doing nothing' cannot possibly be the correct answer*
> *because one does not get marks in a test without doing some work*
> *(much in the same way that 'none of the above' is never the correct*

*option in a multiple choice test!). The fact that they are tempted to 'simplify' this expression in the context of a test question while they would not do so in other contexts means that this item may not be a very good question to use in a test serving a summative or evaluative purpose. However, such considerations do not disqualify the use of such an item for **diagnostic** purposes, because the fact that a student can be 'tricked' into simplifying this expression is relevant information for the teacher, indicating that the understanding of the basic principles of algebra is not secure.*

Wiliam, D., *Integrating formative and summative functions of assessment*

This is not a fair question if you are looking to make a summative inference, but it is a fair one if you are looking to make a formative inference.

A slightly different example will illustrate a similar point. Suppose a teacher has taught a sequence of lessons on the apostrophe of possession and is looking to make a formative inference about whether she can move on to teaching the next topic, or if pupils need some extra work on the apostrophe. Giving pupils a task from a GCSE English writing paper at this point would not allow you to make that inference. GCSE writing papers do assess the mechanics of writing, but they generally require pupils to write extended tasks like letters or stories. This type of assessment allows for a valid summative inference about a pupil's overall writing ability, but it does not allow for a particularly valid formative inference about a pupil's understanding of the apostrophe. Some pupils may write a letter that does not use the apostrophe at all. Others may write a letter that uses the apostrophe of possession correctly three times, and incorrectly three times. Others may write a letter that uses a particularly tricky case of the apostrophe incorrectly, while others may get a simpler case wrong. In short, a GCSE writing task is not a reliable, and therefore not a valid, way to generate a formative inference about whether a pupil has understood the apostrophe of possession.

A sequence of ten multiple-choice questions would be better:

> **Which *three* of these sentences use the apostrophe of possession correctly?**
> **a)** I accidentally dented the mans' car.
> **b)** Jack's cat went missing.
> **c)** The tip of Paige's pencil had broken.
> **d)** The childrens' playground was large and colourful.
> **e)** Tyrone's goal won the match.

Ten questions of this type would give you a much more valid inference about how well pupils have understood the apostrophe, and whether they are ready to move to the next topic. However, it is obviously also the case that these ten questions would not provide you with a valid summative inference about how those pupils are doing relative to their peers. It would not be possible to award a GCSE grade based on them.

Using the same task to provide formative and summative information

We can now return to the question we began this chapter with: to what extent can the same task be used to provide formative and summative information? We can see that the nature of the inference we want to make imposes certain restrictions on the assessment. It may be possible to make some formative inferences from assessments that have been designed for summative purposes, but they will be limited and imperfect in comparison to assessments that have been designed specifically for formative purposes. Similarly, trying to make summative inferences from tasks that have been designed for formative use is hard to do reliably without sacrificing the flexibility and responsiveness of such tasks.

What we see here is the same as we saw in the previous chapter, but from a different angle. Cognitive psychology and assessment theory lead to the same conclusions. The process of acquiring skills is different from the product, and so the methods assessing the process and the product are different too. Cognitive psychology tells us that the end task isn't always helpful for learning, while assessment theory tells us that assessments designed for summative purposes often don't provide valid formative inferences. If we want pupils to develop a certain skill, we have to break that skill down into its component parts and help pupils to acquire the underlying mental model. Similarly, when developing assessments for formative purposes we need to break down the skills and tasks that feature in summative assessments into tasks that will give us valid feedback about how pupils are progressing towards that end goal.

We saw in the previous chapter that programmes like Expressive Writing were able to structure a curriculum so that it broke down the complex skill of writing into a sequence of manageable lessons. It should also be possible to structure an assessment system in the same way and to integrate such an approach to assessment into the curriculum. Indeed, Expressive Writing goes part of the way towards doing this: it is sequenced so that each small activity builds towards the development of a complex skill. As well as this, there are dozens of very flexible and formative assessments in every individual lesson, as well as slightly more structured assessments every 10 lessons which also allow the teacher to judge if he or she needs to reteach any topics. There is no graded summative assessment at the end of the programme, perhaps because the programme is not linked to any national curriculum or national assessment system.

It would be possible to develop a similar programme which did include a summative assessment at the end: a programme that unpicked a complex skill into its constituent parts, sequenced those parts from beginning to end, integrated various formative assessments that allowed teachers to check that their pupils understood, or if any re-teaching was needed, and then included a summative assessment that measured the overall standard achieved at the end of the course. Each of these elements would look quite different, but there would be an overall coherence. When teaching the lesson on ambiguous pronouns, for example, it would be clear to the teacher, and eventually also to the pupil, that whilst the very simple sentence-correction activities looked different to the summative assessment at the end of the unit, those sentence-correction activities were building towards the complex skill and towards the summative assessment measuring that skill. Taken together, a system like this would represent the model of progression we saw Wiliam refer to in the previous chapter: a series of activities that will move pupils 'from their current state to the goal state'.[11]

Thus, even though formative and summative inferences require different types of assessment, it should still be possible to integrate these different assessments into one system. Indeed, this should not only be possible but necessary, as it is by integrating all of these tasks together that the links between them become clearer. If we take this approach, then individual facts can stop being seen as useless information and start to take their place as parts of a larger mental model.

It has to be acknowledged that over the last thirty years, most attempts to create an integrated formative and summative assessment system have not met with great success. In practice, most such systems have required assessments to fulfil several different purposes at once and have excluded tasks which are designed for just one purpose. As we will see, this has led to grades being overused and misused: in particular, attempts to measure formative progress with grades or subgrades has had hugely problematic consequences. Integrating assessments into one system should not mean trying to make different inferences from the same task, nor should it mean grading pupils every lesson. Unfortunately, in practice, this is what has tended to happen.

Part of the reason schools grade pupils frequently is because they are required to do so for accountability purposes. Ofsted does not just judge a school by how its pupils perform in national exams alone: they also request 'the school's own performance information' and 'consider the progress of pupils in **all** year groups, not just those who have taken or are about to take examinations or national tests.'[12] Ofsted does not specify in their handbook how frequent such collections of data need to be, but in 2015, the UK government's Commission on Assessment Without Levels found that many schools were operating assessment systems which required summative data collection every few weeks.[13] A recent Teacher Voice survey commissioned by the Department for Education (DfE) asked 1,920 teachers and senior leaders from 1,549 schools in England the following question: 'Does your school collect data to track pupil progress between statutory and end of key stage assessments?' Figure 3.4 displays their findings.[14]

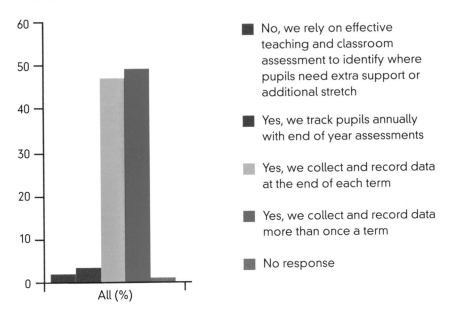

Figure 3.4: Does your school collect data to track pupil progress between statutory and end of key stage assessments? Teacher Voice survey

Only 1% of respondents chose the option: 'No, we rely on effective teaching and classroom assessment to identify where pupils need extra support or additional stretch'. Only 3% said they tracked pupil progress annually. About half said they did so at the end of each term, and half said more frequently than that. This is good evidence that most schools are collecting summative data on their pupils at least three times a year.

In the next two chapters I will outline two popular assessment systems which both aim to provide frequent formative feedback and grades. I will argue that both ultimately fail because they try to draw too many different inferences from the same task. For each system, I will outline how it works and then evaluate it by the validity of the formative and summative inferences it produces. In the final four chapters, I will suggest an integrated model of assessment which might have a better chance of succeeding.

Notes

1 Wiliam, D. and Black, P., 1996. Meanings and Consequences: a basis for distinguishing formative and summative functions of assessment?, *British Educational Research Journal*, 22(5), pp.537–548

2 Koretz, D., 2008. *Measuring up*. Cambridge, Massachusetts: Harvard University Press, pp.30–31

3 *Ibid.* pp.23–28

4 *Ibid.* pp.149–151

5 GL Assessment. *New Group Reading Test Sample Group Progress Report for Teachers* <http://www.gl-assessment.co.uk/sites/gl/files/images/Files/NGRT-Group-progress-report-for-teachers.pdf> accessed 6 November 2016

6 Koretz, 2008, pp.224–225

7 Koretz, D., 1998. Large-scale Portfolio Assessments in the US: evidence pertaining to the quality of measurement, *Assessment in Education: Principles, Policy & Practice*, 5(3), pp.309–334

8 Wiliam, D., 2014. *Principled Assessment Design*. London: SSAT, p.30

9 GL Assessment, 2013. *A Short Guide to Standardised Tests* <http://www.gl-assessment.co.uk/sites/gl/files/images/Guide-to-Standardised-Tests.pdf> accessed 6 November 2016

10 Wiliam, D., 2013. Example of really big mistake: calling formative assessment formative assessment rather than something like "responsive teaching" [Twitter] 23 October <https://twitter.com/dylanwiliam/status/393045049337847808> accessed 6 November 2016

11 Wiliam, D., 2011. *Embedded formative assessment*. Indiana: Solution Tree Press, p.122

12 Ofsted, August 2015. *School inspection handbook: Handbook for inspecting schools in England under section 5 of the Education Act 2005*, p.54

13 Department for Education, 2015. *Final Report on the Commission on Assessment without Levels*, p.31 <https://www.gov.uk/government/uploads/system/uploads/attachment_data/file/483058/Commission_on_Assessment_Without_Levels_-_report.pdf> accessed 6 November 2016

14 Straw, S., Tattersall, J. and Sims, D., 2016. *NFER Teacher voice omnibus: Research report*. London: Department for Education, p.17 <https://www.gov.uk/government/uploads/system/uploads/attachment_data/file/535269/DFE-RR532-Teacher-voice-omnibus-November-2015-responses.pdf> accessed 6 November 2016

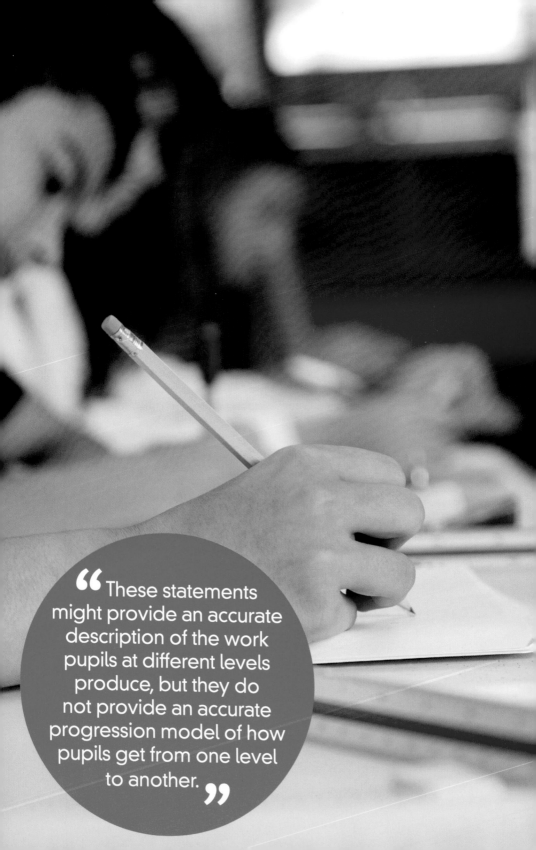

These statements might provide an accurate description of the work pupils at different levels produce, but they do not provide an accurate progression model of how pupils get from one level to another.

Descriptor-based assessment 4

How does this model work?

One way of combining the formative and summative purposes of assessments is to use descriptors of performance. Teachers can use these descriptors to assess pupils' work in individual lessons. Then, at the end of a set period of time, all of these lesson-by-lesson judgements can be aggregated to provide a summative grade. In an ideal world, one might be able to get rid of a lot of formal summative examinations and replace them with frequent collections of formative information.

There have been many different practical manifestations of this approach. In England, National Curriculum levels were developed at the same time as the National Curriculum in the late 1980s and consisted of statements of attainment at different levels.[1] As we've seen, they were only meant to be used for summative purposes at the end of phases of education. However, as we have also seen, it was possible for them to be used more frequently than that. In 2008, the English government introduced the Assessing Pupils' Progress (APP) scheme, which was based on National Curriculum levels and was explicitly designed to be used very frequently.[2] A central part of this scheme was the APP grid: a detailed A3 sheet of paper which broke down a subject into certain assessment focuses and then provided descriptions of achievement at each level within each focus. For example, the writing APP grid had eight assessment focuses with eight levels each. One assessment focus was that pupils should 'write imaginative, interesting and thoughtful texts', and to get the top level on this focus, a pupil had to display 'creative selection and adaptation of a wide range of forms and conventions to meet varied writing challenges with distinctive personal voice and style matched to intended effect'.[3]

Although National Curriculum levels and APP are no longer a part of government policy, a number of subsequent systems have adopted a very similar approach. In fact, the government's temporary replacement for National Curriculum levels at primary level, the interim frameworks, are also based on descriptions of performance.[4] Other educational organisations have filled the gap left by National Curriculum levels with very similar systems.

The National Association of Head Teachers (NAHT) have proposed a system of Key Performance Indicators (KPIs).[5] Pearson have a set of Progression Frameworks consisting of descriptions of performance at different levels in Key Stage 3.[6] Classroom Monitor have developed a tracking system which can be populated with different sets of statements, one of which is the NAHT KPI system, and another of which is APP.[7] Herts for Learning's replacement for levels also consists of a similar set of statements, as does the one developed by Target Tracker, which 'breaks the new curriculum into easy-to-understand statements'.[8-9] These systems are widespread: every state primary school has to use the interim frameworks as they are a part of statutory assessment, whilst Target Tracker is used by approximately 4,000 primaries and Classroom monitor by approximately 2,000 (as of September 2016).[10-11] The chart in Figure 4.1 compares the type of statements found in these different systems.

Comparison of example statements found in different assessment systems

Assessment system	Example statement	Possible levels or grades
National Curriculum levels	Pupils show creativity in the way they select specific features or expressions to convey effects and to interest the reader	1–8, and 'exceptional performance'
Assessing Pupils' Progress (APP)	Organise and present whole texts effectively, sequencing and structuring information, ideas and events	1–8, divided into low, secure and high or c / b / a
National curriculum interim frameworks for teacher assessments	The pupil can write for a range of purposes and audiences: managing shifts between levels of formality through selecting vocabulary precisely and by manipulating grammatical structures	Working towards the expected standard, working at the expected standard, working at greater depth within the expected standard
National Association of Head Teachers Key Performance Indicators	Identifies the audience for, and purpose of, the writing	1 - working below expectations, 2 - working at the expected level, 3 - working beyond expectations
Herts for Learning	Evaluates the effectiveness of own and others' writing and suggests improvements	Entering, developing, securing, deepening
Target Tracker Steps Framework	Evaluate and edit by assessing the effectiveness of his/her own and others' writing with reasoning	b = beginning b+ = beginning plus w = working within w+ = working within plus s = secure s+ = secure plus

Figure 4.1: Example statements found in assessment systems.[12]

In each of these systems, the teacher uses these statements in individual lessons to assess each pupil's performance. Most of these systems also recommend that teachers share the statements, or pupil-friendly versions of the statements, with pupils so they can monitor and assess their own progress. The Qualifications and Curriculum Development Authority (QCDA) suggested giving pupils their own A3 APP grid which they could highlight as they progressed.[13] Herts for Learning recommend that when using their current assessment system, the 'key to talking to a child is…to focus on the criteria', whilst in the past they also developed a set of 'pupil-friendly' criteria for APP.[8,14] An early evaluation of APP showed that it encouraged teachers to use the language of the grids in the feedback they gave to pupils.[15] The Target Tracker Steps Framework provides pupil-friendly statements as part of the package: so, for instance, the statement 'Provide reasoned justifications for his/her views' is simplified to 'I can fully explain my views with reasons and evidence from the text.' These pupil-friendly statements are available as sheets that can be stuck into the front of pupils' books for easy reference.[16]

Once the statements have been used in individual lessons to assess performance, the teacher can then aggregate all these judgements and use them to create a summative grade. As Classroom Monitor puts it, this allows for 'summative results [to be] populated from the formative assessment markbook'.[17] Exactly how this aggregation is to be made is a source of some difficulty. Should a pupil have to meet all of the statements at a particular level, or just some of them, in order to achieve that particular level?

To help solve this difficulty, a number of these systems feature some kind of algorithm or formula which allows teachers to derive a grade from their lesson-by-lesson judgements against the various levels. This approach dates right back to the very earliest days of National Curriculum levels, when one method of adding up formative judgements was proposed by the Schools Examination and Assessment Council: 'This rule suggested that where there were one or two statements of attainment at a particular level in an attainment target, all had to be attained in order for the student to be awarded that level, and where there were three or more statements, all but one had to be attained.'[18] Similarly, Assessing Pupils' Progress for Reading at Key Stage 3 came with this guidance:

> **For level 2:** ticks at level 2 for AF1, AF2 and some highlighting at level 2 for AF3.
> **For level 3:** ticks at level 3 for AF2, AF3 and one other AF out of AFs 1, 4, 5, 6, 7.
> AF1 is not assessed separately beyond level 3.
> **For level 4:** ticks at level 4 for AF2 and AF3 and at least one other AF.
> **For level 5:** ticks at level 5 for any four AFs provided there is at least level 4 for AF3.
>
> Department for Children, Schools and Families (DCSF):
> *APP Assessment Criteria: Reading*

The APP guidance, however, also stressed that such advice should not be seen as a mathematical formula, but more as a support for professional judgement.[19] Many of the newer models feature similar guidance that is designed to be used in a more systematic way. The NAHT have a spreadsheet to accompany their statements which calculates a pupil's overall standard based on what their teacher enters for each individual statement.[5] Herts for Learning recommend that pupils should meet 25% of the statements in order to be judged 'entering', 60% in order to be 'developing', 80% in order to be 'securing' and all, or almost all, in order to be 'deepening'.[8] The Target Tracker Steps Framework, meanwhile, takes a graphic approach: 'To monitor pupil progression within statements, mark tick boxes when attainment levels have been met, e.g. one tick box for 'Working Towards' and a second for 'Achieved'. To monitor overall pupil progression within the subject, colour in the progression bar at the top of the page using a highlighter pen.'[16]

These different systems have different names for the standards pupils can achieve. Some have eight or nine levels, others have three or four labels like 'entering' or 'emerging'. Although they all have different names, in essence all of these categories involve making a summative judgement. As we saw in the previous chapter, every time we sum up a pupil's performance with one of these levels or labels, we are making a judgement about how pupils are doing in the summative sense. We are trying to create a shared meaning. Even if we did not mean the assessment to be a summative one, the moment we use a grade, a level, or a value-laden statement or word, we are making a summative inference. In order for that summative inference to be reliable, the assessment it is based on needs to follow all the restrictions outlined in Chapter 3: it has to be taken in standard conditions, distinguish between candidates and sample from a broad domain. If it doesn't, the risk is that we are telling pupils and ourselves things that are simply wrong.

This is especially, although not only, the case when we use grades or labels which are also used for national assessments: such grades are used in formal national assessments to mean things about how pupils do compared to every pupil nationally. We cannot use them in the classroom to mean something completely different to how they are used nationally. Similar restrictions apply to words like 'emerging' and 'exceeding' because such words have an everyday shared meaning. Every time we make a summative inference, we are making a significant claim that requires a high standard of evidence to justify it. If we make that claim without the right standard of evidence, there is a good chance the claim will be wrong.

To sum up, these systems consist of a set of descriptors of different levels of performance. Teachers use these formatively in individual lessons to help plan and give feedback to pupils. Then, at the end of a certain period of time, they aggregate these judgements and use a formula to calculate the summative standard a pupil has reached. In the rest of this chapter we'll consider first, if this model provides valid formative data and second, if it provides valid summative data.

Does this model provide valid formative data?

It's difficult to get valid formative information from a descriptor-based model for three reasons: these models are based around descriptions of, not analysis of, performance; they are generic models, which means they lack the useful specificity we've looked at in previous chapters; they do not allow teachers to assess the difference between fleeting performance and genuine long-term learning.

Descriptive, not analytic

Descriptor-based models are, as their name would suggest, based on descriptions of performance at different levels. They are not based on the analysis of what causes performance. As a result, if they are used formatively, they place focus on holistic and complex performances rather than the specific and isolated components of such performances. This is true of all subjects, but it is particularly the case for reading. This is because the models presented by these descriptors are especially different from the way we know that reading skill develops. As such, it's worth looking more closely at a set of reading descriptors to illustrate the wider point about the differences between analysis and description.

The following eight descriptors are taken from an APP reading grid. Although these grids have now been discontinued, they are quite similar in style to the new government interim frameworks and the reading descriptors produced by the systems we looked at earlier in this chapter. The grid describes performance from a level 1 to a level 8 on one particular assessment focus: Assessment Focus 3 (AF3), 'deduce, infer or interpret information, events or ideas from texts'.

In some reading, usually with support: reasonable inference at a basic level; comments/questions about meanings of parts of texts

In some reading: simple, plausible inference about events and information, using evidence from text; comments based on textual cues, sometimes misunderstood

In most reading: straightforward inference based on a single point of reference in the text; responses to text show meaning established at a literal level

Across a range of reading: comments make inferences based on evidence from different points in the text; inferences often correct, but comments are not always rooted securely in the text or repeat narrative or content

Across a range of reading: comments develop explanation of inferred meanings drawing on evidence across the text; comments make inferences and deductions based on textual evidence

Across a range of reading: comments securely based in textual evidence and identify different layers of meaning, with some attempt at detailed exploration of them; comments consider wider implications or significance of information, events or ideas in the text

Across a range of reading: comments begin to develop an interpretation of the text(s), making connections between insights, teasing out meanings or weighing up evidence

Across a range of reading: clear critical stance develops a coherent interpretation of text(s), drawing on imaginative insights and well supported by reference and wider textual knowledge

Department for Children, Schools and Families (DCSF):
APP Assessment guidelines: Reading

These descriptors are clearly designed to assess final performance against complex tasks: in this case, performance on a comprehension task. But, as we saw in Chapter 2, a pupil's ability to 'deduce, infer or interpret information, events or ideas from texts' is dependent on a broad range of knowledge. The activities that would help a pupil progress from making 'reasonable inferences at a basic level' up to developing 'a coherent interpretation of text(s), drawing on imaginative insights and well supported by reference and wider textual knowledge' may not necessarily involve practising making inferences and imaginative insights. Instead, pupils may benefit from a variety of different tasks which could not be measured in this way. These statements might provide an accurate description of the work pupils at different levels produce, but they do not provide an accurate progression model of how pupils get from one level to another.

What would an accurate reading progression model look like? Inference, or being able to read between the lines, is a vital part of reading and the ability to make sophisticated inferences is one of the things that marks out better readers. But what causes some pupils to be able to make better inferences than others? Is it that they have had more practice and experience at inferring? Or is it something else? Reading research shows that a pupil's vocabulary and the extent of their background knowledge make a huge difference to their ability to infer meaning from texts.[20] The following sentence uses fairly straightforward vocabulary, but is hard to comprehend without a specific piece of background knowledge:

> I believed John when he said he had a lake house, until he said it was forty feet from the water at high tide.
>
> Willingham, D.T., *Why Don't Students Like School?*, p.31

When they read this sentence, many pupils – and indeed adults – stare at it in confusion. The key piece of background knowledge needed to make sense of it is that lakes do not have appreciable tides. Once you know that, the sentence makes sense, and it is possible to start to 'develop an interpretation of the text(s), making connections between insights, teasing out meanings or weighing up evidence.' When you know that lakes don't have appreciable tides, you can infer that John is a boastful and materialistic individual who lies about his wealth. If you don't know that lakes don't have appreciable tides, that inference is not possible.

Something similar is true for vocabulary. When reading a text, we need to know the meaning of 95% of the words in a text: anything below this and our understanding starts to break down.[21] Many teachers will be familiar with the experience of otherwise good readers struggling with a new text that requires knowledge of an obscure or unfamiliar word. For example, one GCSE examiner's report mentions how many pupils struggled with an unseen comprehension that required knowledge of the word 'glacier'.[22]

Given the importance of vocabulary, it is worth teaching it explicitly. In *Bringing Words to Life: Robust Vocabulary Instruction*, the reading researchers Isabel Beck, Margaret G. McKeown and Linda Kucan outline the research on vocabulary instruction and recommend a series of practical activities which can help to build a pupil's vocabulary. Among the activities they recommend are questions and quizzes like the following:[23]

Which would be easier to notice?
- A house all alone on a hill or a house crowded in with lots of other buildings?
- A barking dog or a dog sleeping on a porch?
- An ant crawling along the floor or a snake slithering along the floor?

Which would plod?

- Frankenstein in a castle or a ghost in a castle?
- A huge dinosaur or a mountain lion?
- A heavy man or a skinny man?
- A girl who was really tired or a girl in a race?

Any model of how pupils make progress in reading, therefore, has to recognise the development of vocabulary and allow for the use of the kinds of activities and assessments recommended by Beck and others. This is because acquiring vocabulary leads to pupils being able to make more sophisticated inferences.

If we look at the descriptor-based models of reading outlined earlier, we can see that it would be extremely hard to assess performance on the tasks Beck and her co-authors recommend using such descriptors. Suppose a pupil successfully answered ten vocabulary questions like the ones shown. That would not be sufficient evidence to conclude that the pupil was a level 1, or a level 4 at inferring information, or whether they were 'emerging' or 'expected' in their inference skills. Similarly, if a pupil was described as being a level 4 at inferring information, it would not give you much useful information about whether they had or had not learnt a series of new words in a lesson.

In short, the descriptors would not tell you if pupils had done well or badly on a set of questions about vocabulary. And that set of vocabulary questions would not tell you if pupils had reached a certain descriptor or not. The descriptors in the assessment framework are simply not compatible with certain types of questions. Ultimately, these descriptors are best suited to describing summative performance, and they are therefore best matched to tasks that have been designed in order to produce such a summative shared meaning.

In the previous chapter, we outlined three important features assessments need in order to produce such shared meanings: they need to be completed in standard and comparable conditions by all the pupils taking it; they have to consist of questions of moderate difficulty that distinguish between the pupils taking the assessment; and they have to sample from a wide domain. For the descriptors in the previous paragraphs, the best kind of task for generating this shared meaning would be an unseen reading passage followed by a set of questions. In general, reading assessments tend to consist of such tasks. However, an unseen comprehension is not good at providing formative information about a pupil's strengths, weaknesses and what they should do next to improve. As we've seen, a pupil can struggle to make an accurate inference about a text, but this could be to do with a lack of background knowledge or of key vocabulary. It is also not always clear from a pupil's response exactly what knowledge or vocabulary is lacking.

We have looked closely here at how reading descriptors work, but the same reasoning applies to other subjects. Indeed, in subjects where exams require a lot of reading, exactly the same reasoning about the importance of vocabulary applies: a pupil may find it difficult to answer a history source question because of unfamiliar vocabulary. Even in subjects like maths and science, the same general principle applies. If a pupil is struggling with a complex task, it can be hard to work out exactly why they are struggling, and therefore hard to provide them with specific and useful feedback. Descriptors encourage complex tasks, discourage focussed tasks, and so make it harder to give useful feedback.

It might be argued that this type of assessment system does not actually stop teachers from using certain tasks; teachers are free to use whatever activities they want in lessons as long as they realise that only some of them are capable of contributing to the final grade. However, the advice accompanying such systems does favour certain activities.

Guides to APP explicitly recommended that teachers should stop using focused and specific tasks, and start using broader and more complex ones. For example, one guide recommended that teachers use more problem-solving tasks to teach and assess maths, and that they move away from 'using spelling tests' and towards 'making some assessments of spelling across a range of writing'.[24]

Not only do such systems explicitly warn against using certain types of tasks, but most of them are designed to be used every lesson and require judgements to be made about hundreds of different statements, which means there is no time left to do anything that doesn't fit into the system. These systems are also set up to allow for very frequent grading, which further increases the pressure on the activities being used in each lesson. The Assessing Pupils' Progress handbook did recommend that this system was to be used to produce summative levels no more than three times a year.[25] However, there is plenty of evidence to suggest that APP resulted in pupils being given a level at the end of every lesson. Some of the newer assessment systems even encourage this because they allow for 'live' updating of summative grades, so that every time a teacher updates the formative grid, the summative grade can be correspondingly updated too.[17]

This puts enormous pressure on the activities in individual lessons to be the kinds of restrictive, complex and holistic tasks that one can derive a grade from. Indeed, what can very often happen in these cases is that tasks like spelling tests or vocabulary quizzes get a bad reputation. This is because they do not provide very good evidence for the final grade and, compared to larger and more complex tasks, they can seem quite trivial, basic and as though they are not stretching pupils.

I can remember being given this advice after setting a class a spelling test where the pupils all got 8 or more out of 10. The problem with this test, I was told, was that it did not allow pupils to demonstrate fully what they were capable of. And indeed, it was true that this class were capable of doing much, much more than spelling 8 or 9 words correctly. But, if every lesson is set up to allow pupils to demonstrate fully what they are capable of, then lessons start to look less like lessons and more like exams. This is the logic of descriptor-based assessment systems: every lesson has to generate evidence that can be used to describe a pupil's overall performance, and so the outcome is that every lesson starts to look like an exam.

Generic, not specific

Second, as well as being descriptive, not analytic, this approach is a generic one that does not take into account the specific detail within each subject. All of the descriptors and statements we have looked at are generic: that is, they could be applied to any kind of content. Indeed, that was often seen as a strength of levels: they applied a similar abstract model to all subjects, showing that the underlying progression from lower to higher order skills was consistent across subjects. For example, the reading descriptors we just looked at do not mention any specific literary texts and the old National Curriculum history level descriptors do not mention any specific historical eras. Feedback based on such descriptors was therefore unable to be precise or specific. This might not be a problem if the descriptors were not used to produce feedback and targets, but as we saw at the start of this chapter, these systems encourage teachers to use the language of the generic descriptors with pupils.

A couple of examples will show just how helpful specific feedback can be, and how unhelpful generic feedback can be. Take the following, relatively simple, question:

Who did William defeat at the Battle of Hastings?

The correct answer is Harold Godwinson, but suppose a pupil replies with 'Harald Hardrada'. This answer allows teachers to provide some very useful feedback. They could direct the pupil to reread the section in the textbook about the Battle of Hastings and then ask the pupil to answer the question again. If enough pupils made the same mistake, the teacher could replan the start of the next lesson to address this misunderstanding by retelling the story of 1066 with a specific focus on Harald Hardrada and Harold Godwinson. Or, the teacher could simply say to the pupil: 'You've confused Harold Godwinson and Harald Hardrada.'

As we have seen, such a question is less likely to be asked within a descriptor-based assessment system. Instead, a pupil is more likely to get a question that can be graded. For example, perhaps a piece of extended writing on the following question: 'In your opinion, in 1066 which of the three contenders to the throne of England had the best claim?' A pupil may well still be confused about the identity of the three claimants, and if that is the case, she will probably write a fairly confused essay. However, the teacher will find it much more difficult to establish the source of the confusion, because the essay will involve so much else. Even if it is obvious that the pupil has confused two of the claimants, the teacher won't be able to correct the misconception clearly if feedback is given on the basis of the generic descriptors. Instead, they will end up saying something like 'your knowledge of the past is emerging, but it is not yet developing'. Clearly, it is far more helpful and specific to be told that 'You've confused Harald Hardrada and Harold Godwinson' than to be told that 'You've displayed an emerging knowledge of the past, but in order to improve, you need to develop your knowledge of the past.'

This pupil's misunderstanding is about something that is quite basic and straightforward to correct. But even at more advanced levels of understanding, there is still value in isolating the different components of a task and, even at these advanced levels, essays are not necessarily the best way of working out how a pupil needs to improve. Take the following question, for example.

> **Why was Stalin able to defeat Trotsky in the struggle for power in the Soviet Union?**
>
> **a)** Stalin had been chosen by Lenin as the next leader.
> **b)** Stalin supported the popular policy of world revolution.
> **c)** Stalin controlled appointments in the Communist Party.
> **d)** Stalin had gained support from the Red Army by leading it in the Revolution.

This question is taken from a Canadian history exam designed to be taken by 17-year-old school leavers, but it could be used in the classroom and accompanied with feedback.[26] Because it is a multiple-choice question, it allows the teacher to give very specific feedback: each of the incorrect options has been designed to target a specific misconception. This question could easily be adapted to become an essay question which was marked using descriptors. However, it would be harder to get such useful feedback from an essay as well as harder to communicate the feedback using descriptors.

The problem with feedback from descriptors is not one that can be solved by rewriting them in 'pupil-friendly' language. A target can be written in words that a pupil can understand, but can still be unhelpful. For example, the following is taken from a pupil-friendly set of descriptors:

> I can make simple, plausible best guesses about events and information in a text and I can identify the simple, most obvious points although I sometimes get confused if points are made in different places in a text.
>
> Herts Grid for Learning, *Student-Friendly APP Reading Assessment Focuses*

It is a rewrite of the following from the APP Assessment Criteria for Reading:

> **Level 2:** simple, plausible inferences about events and information, using evidence from text and comments based on textual cues.
> **Level 3:** straightforward inference based on a single point of reference in the text.
>
> DCSF, *APP Assessment guidelines: Reading*

The first statement does use some simpler words than the second, but it is not much more helpful. Ensuring that a pupil can understand a target and act on it involves thinking about not just the words in the target, but also how well the pupil's own mental models are developed. For example, I can remember writing the target 'use more full stops' on a piece of work. On the surface, this seems quite a specific target which a pupil could understand and act on. Most Secondary pupils would understand what that meant, and would be able to take action in response to it. But that does not mean it would definitely help them to improve. If a pupil's understanding of sentence structure was very well-developed, and she had missed out full stops as a result of carelessness, then the target would be helpful. But if her problem was that she was using lots of run-on sentences because her understanding of sentence structures was very weak, then such a target would not be helpful at all, because she would not know where she should be using more full stops.

A colleague of mine once parodied these kinds of targets by saying that it would be better to write: 'Well done, you've used full stops. Next time, try to use them correctly.' In order to know how to use full stops correctly, pupils need to be able to identify sentences, and to do that, they need to be able to recognise subjects and verbs. That is why the Expressive Writing programme begins by teaching pupils what subjects and verbs are, because it recognises that this is what allows pupils to write accurate sentences.

It's often said that one of the advantages of a descriptor-based model is that it allows pupils to engage with what is expected of them and to understand clearly what their next steps are. But when the descriptors are so generic, this is not true. Generic targets provide the illusion of clarity: they seem like they are providing feedback, but they are actually much more like grades. Research shows that when pupils receive a grade and a comment on a piece of work, they are less likely to focus on the comment and more likely to focus on their grade, and the grades of their peers.[27] As a result, in order to get pupils to pay attention to the comment, it's best to leave out the grade. However, if the comment is descriptive rather than analytic, then it is effectively grade-like in its function: that is, it is accurate but not helpful. Leaving out the grade may mean the pupil will focus more on the comment, but if the comment is not providing any more helpful information than the grade, it is not going to help the pupil improve. In fact, descriptor-based comments are effectively just grades in prose.

Short-term, not long-term

The third reason why such models fail to provide good formative feedback is that they do not offer a means of distinguishing between short-term performance and long-term learning. In Chapter 1 we saw that the definition of learning is 'a change in long-term memory', and that as a result, a good performance doesn't guarantee pupils have learnt something: 'that performance is often fleeting and, consequently, a highly imperfect index of learning does not appear to be appreciated by learners or instructors who frequently misinterpret short-term performance as a guide to long-term learning.'[28]

Arguably, the most difficult factor in establishing reliable formative inferences is the difference between short-term performance and long-term learning. This is because often we want to make such inferences immediately, in the middle of a lesson, or soon after the end, so we can make a quick decision about what to do next. Yet, if we want to make an inference about whether a pupil needs more teaching on a topic, or if they are ready to move on, then a formative assessment which takes place soon after the lesson cannot allow us to make such an inference.

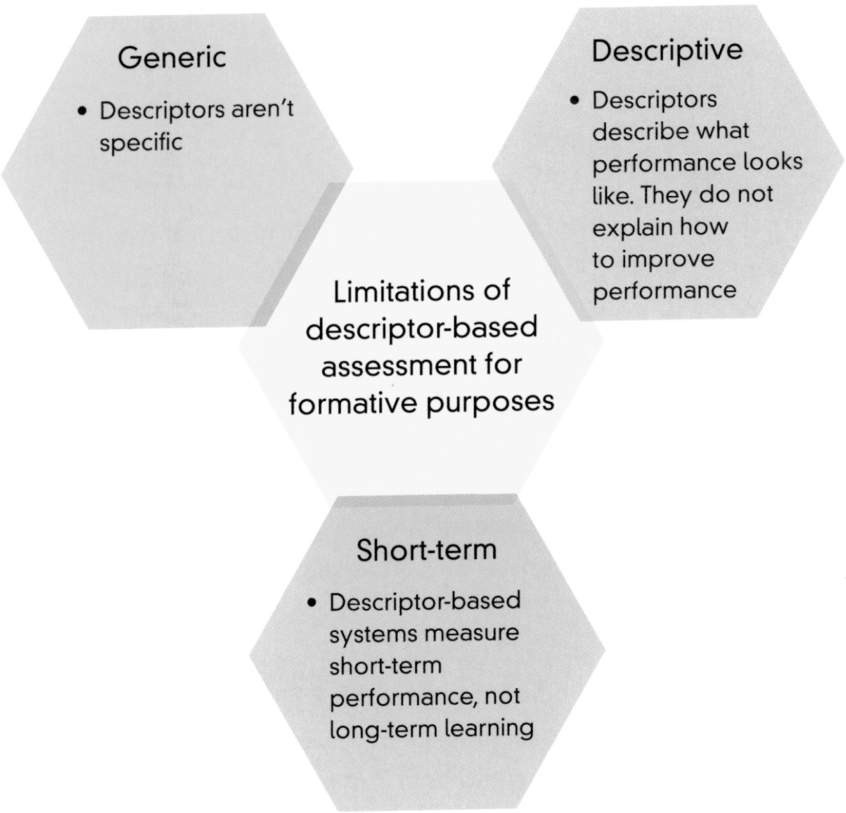

Generic

- Descriptors aren't specific

Descriptive

- Descriptors describe what performance looks like. They do not explain how to improve performance

Limitations of descriptor-based assessment for formative purposes

Short-term

- Descriptor-based systems measure short-term performance, not long-term learning

Figure 4.2: Limitations of descriptor-based assessment for formative purposes

The only possible solution here is to supplement our formative inferences with information about the typical time it takes for pupils to learn something new. Even if a whole class of pupils get every single question right at the end of a lesson, the teacher should not assume that the class need no further work on this topic. These descriptor-based systems do not account for the difference between performance and learning. In the case of maths, for example, one of the APP statements is 'recall multiplication facts up to 10 × 10 and quickly derive corresponding division facts'.[29] It's entirely possible that a pupil might be able to do this at the end of a unit of work, but that they have still not learnt it securely. There is no way of making this distinction within these systems.

Does this model provide valid summative data?

There are three main reasons why it is difficult to get valid summative data from a descriptor-based model. First, it is based around judgements against prose descriptors, and such judgements are hard to do reliably. Second, the model is based on work done in lessons, not in formal assessment conditions, which means that pupils are not being treated consistently. This, too, makes it hard to make reliable judgements. Third, these systems depend to a great degree on teacher judgement. Whilst teacher judgement offers some advantages over formal exams, it also introduces problems with bias and stereotypes.

Judgements against prose descriptors

The descriptor-based model involves making judgements against prose descriptors. Making accurate judgements against such descriptors feels as though it should be straightforward, but in actual fact, it leads to very significant difficulties because it is possible to interpret such statements in very different ways. Let's look at an example given in Wiliam's *Principled Assessment Design*. Consider the prose statement: 'Can compare two fractions to identify which is larger'.[30]

This feels quite specific and precise. But it is possible to create hundreds of questions that are all legitimate interpretations of that statement. And many of those questions will be of varying difficulty. Consider the following three questions:

> Which is bigger: $\frac{3}{7}$ or $\frac{5}{7}$?
> Which is bigger: $\frac{3}{4}$ or $\frac{4}{5}$?
> Which is bigger: $\frac{5}{7}$ or $\frac{5}{9}$?

These three questions all involve comparing two fractions to identify which is larger. But pupils do not find them all equally difficult. 90% of English 14-year-olds got the first question right. Only 75% got the second one right. And only 15% got the last one right. Imagine a group of teachers attempting to decide if their pupils have met this statement or not on the basis of classwork. Even slight differences in the types of questions the teachers have asked will make a huge difference to their decision.

Paul Bambrick-Santoyo, a charter school leader in the USA, has made a similar point. He cites a maths descriptor that is taken from New Jersey's Grade 7 content standards: 'Understand and use ratios, proportions and percents in a variety of situations.'[31]

He then lists six questions, which are all completely legitimate interpretations of that descriptor:

1. Identify 50% of 20.
2. Identify 67% of 81.
3. Shawn got 7 correct answers out of 10 possible answers on his science test. What percent of questions did he get correct?

4. JJ Redick was on pace to set an NCAA record in career free throw percentage. Leading into the NCAA tournament in 2004, he made 97 of 104 free throw attempts. What percentage of free throws did he make?

5. JJ Redick was on pace to set an NCAA record in career free throw percentage. Leading into the NCAA tournament in 2004, he made 97 of 104 free throw attempts. In his first tournament game, Redick missed his first five free throws. How far did his percentage drop from before the tournament game to right after missing those free throws?

6. JJ Redick and Chris Paul were competing for the best free-throw shooting percentage. Redick made 94% of his first 103 shots, while Paul made 47 out of 51 shots.

   a) Which one had a better shooting percentage?

   b) In the next game, Redick made only 2 of 10 shots while Paul made 7 of 10 shots. What are their new overall shooting percentages? Who is the better shooter?

   c) Jason argued that if Paul and JJ each made their next ten shots, their shooting percentages would go up the same amount. Is this true? Why or why not?

Whilst each question is a legitimate interpretation of the descriptor, they 'differ tremendously in scope, difficulty and design'.[31] If six different teachers were to use these six different questions to assess how well their class were doing on this descriptor, their results would not be comparable at all. Such a process cannot produce a shared meaning.

The two maths descriptors in the previous paragraph are about as precise and objective as it is possible for descriptors to be, and yet they are still capable of many different interpretations. In other subjects, the problems are even greater. Take English, for example. Confronted with a statement like 'identify and comment on the structure and organisation of texts, including grammatical and presentational features at text level', one teacher could choose to teach a unit on 19th-century novels where most of the classwork consisted of lengthy written answers, while another could choose to teach a unit on modern poetry where most of the classwork consisted of annotated posters.[32] Comparing performance on one of these tasks with performance on another is enormously difficult.

Not only does this make it difficult to compare pupils in different classes and schools, but it also makes it difficult to compare the same pupils over time. Many English teachers using this system faced a problem when assessing pupils' work on Shakespeare: pupils got persistently lower levels when studying Shakespeare than on other units. Pupils who were able to show clear understanding and critical evaluation (a level 8 skill) when writing an essay about a modern novel such as *Holes*, by Louis Sachar, were unable to meet such a standard when studying *A Midsummer Night's Dream*. Of course, this is not surprising: regardless of the cultural value of the two texts, *A Midsummer Night's Dream* is technically more difficult than most modern novels. Simply understanding the plot of *A Midsummer Night's Dream* is therefore arguably as technically demanding as analysing a modern novel. However, the set of generic descriptors suggests that the skill of analysis is constant, and that therefore a pupil who is unable to analyse a Shakespearean text in as much detail as a modern novel has regressed.

At least in the case of the maths descriptors examples ('Can compare two fractions to identify which is larger' and 'Understand and use ratios, proportions and percents in a variety of situations'), once the question had been created it was straightforward to tell if a pupil had got it right or wrong. In the case of quality-model assessments such as essays, the descriptors were not only used to devise the task, but they were used to mark it too. Ensuring that different markers interpret a statement like 'a wide ranging vocabulary used imaginatively and with precision' in the same way is also extremely difficult. As a result of all of these problems, it is perhaps no surprise that many of the studies that have been carried out on this style of assessment report very low levels of reliability.[33]

One possible response to this problem is to write descriptors that are more precise and less capable of different interpretations. However, this is not as simple as it sounds, and many attempts to do this have ended in failure. As Professor Alison Wolf of King's College London says, 'one cannot, either in principle or in theory, develop written descriptors so tight that they can be applied reliably, by multiple assessors, to multiple assessment situations.'[34] Words are not always as good at communicating meaning as we assume. The philosophers of science, Michael Polanyi and Thomas Kuhn, wrote extensively on this issue.[35-36] In *Second Thoughts on Paradigms*, Kuhn addresses almost exactly this problem when discussing the way the typical science textbook works:

> *Students of physics regularly report that they have read through a chapter of their text, understood it perfectly, but nonetheless had difficulty solving the problems at the end of the chapter. Almost invariably their difficulty is in setting up the appropriate equations, in relating the words and examples given in the text to the particular problems they are asked to solve.*
>
> Kuhn, T.S., *Second Thoughts on Paradigms*, p.305

For Kuhn, the solution to this problem is not textbooks that are better written, or words that have more precise definitions. For him, the solution is the 'problem-set' or series of exercises at the end of each textbook chapter:

> *In the course of their training a vast number of such exercises are set for them, and students entering the same specialty regularly do very*

nearly the same ones…These concrete problems with their solutions
are what I previously referred to as exemplars, a community's standard
examples…Acquiring an arsenal of exemplars…is integral to the
process by which a student gains access to the cognitive achievements
of his disciplinary group. Without exemplars he would never learn
much of what the group knows about such fundamental concepts as
force and field, element and compound, or nucleus and cell.

Kuhn, T.S., *Second Thoughts on Paradigms*, p.305

Complex concepts such as 'force', 'element' and 'compound' are not actually given meaning through prose definition. Instead, they are defined through examples. Similarly, defining performance through written descriptors will never be precise enough. Instead, we need exemplars: either examples of actual tasks that pupils have to solve, or of actual pupil work. We'll consider these solutions more in the final chapter, as finding replacements for imprecise prose descriptors is one of the most important parts of an assessment system.

Differing work conditions

We've seen that one problem with the descriptor-based model is the lack of specificity of the descriptors, and the inconsistency this causes. The second problem is the inconsistency caused by differing conditions. The descriptor-based model asks teachers to make formative judgements in lessons and then aggregate them into a summative judgement. However, the problem is that in each lesson pupils will have completed tasks in very different conditions. Again, subtle differences in how a task is presented will have a big impact on a pupil's ability to do the task. For example, a pupil's understanding could be affected if one teacher reads a poem out loud whilst another asks pupils to read it to each other. If one teacher supplies a follow-up prompting question, and another does not, that too will affect the pupil's answer. Two pupils may have produced very similar work: a page in their maths book full of correct answers to questions, or an essay of similar quality in their English exercise book, but if one pupil produced the work independently, and another was given prompts by a teacher, then it is not fair to compare them. Just looking at the final piece of work does not tell you about the conditions the work was completed in, which makes using the work alone to generate a summative judgement very unreliable.

One attempt to solve these problems of inconsistency is the algorithm, or formula, we saw at the start of this chapter. This applied a standard procedure to all the different evidence collected by different teachers. The problem with this kind of formula is that it just papered over the genuine and irreconcilable differences in how the judgements about each statement were arrived at. The surface precision of such algorithms gave an appearance of rigour and comparability to data that was essentially not comparable. Applying a consistent formula to inconsistent data will not lead to consistent results. An anecdote told by Charles Babbage expresses this point well. Babbage invented one of the first calculators, and told the following story about how people responded to the invention:

> *On two occasions I have been asked, — "Pray, Mr. Babbage, if you put into the machine wrong figures, will the right answers come out?" I am not able rightly to apprehend the kind of confusion of ideas that could provoke such a question.*
>
> Babbage, C., *Passages from the Life of a Philosopher*, p.67

If the data entered into a system is not comparable, applying a standard algorithm to it will not make it comparable.

Bias and stereotyping

The third and final problem with this model is that of bias and stereotyping. The descriptor-based model relies heavily on teacher judgement. This was supposed to solve one of the pervasive problems which causes unreliability in exam results: the problem of the variability of student performance on the day. This is one of the biggest sources of exam unreliability, and one of the hardest to eliminate; every teacher knows how frustrating it can be when a pupil gets an exam grade that is not a true reflection of their ability. Often, this happens because pupils have good days and bad days when they do the exam. Relying more on teacher judgement promises to solve this problem by involving the people who know pupils best in the assessment procedure: teachers.

However, whilst teachers certainly know pupils best, they are also subject – as all humans are – to bias. It is a well-established but poorly recognised fact: teacher assessment is biased against disadvantaged pupils. Again and again, study after study shows that teachers tend to mark down pupils from ethnic minorities, pupils from lower-income backgrounds, pupils with special educational needs, and pupils with behavioural problems.[37–41] When researchers compare the scores such pupils get in teacher assessments with the scores they get on exams, they find that teachers persistently undermark them.

Such bias is not conscious, and it is not particular to teachers; rather, it happens because of a weakness all humans have in making complex judgements.[42] That is to say, teacher assessment is biased not because it is carried out by teachers, but because it is carried out by humans. Tammy Campbell, an Institute of Education researcher whose recent research showed bias in teacher assessments of 7-year-olds, is at pains to point this out. She says: 'I want to stress that this isn't something unique to teachers. It's human nature. Humans use stereotypes as a cognitive shortcut and we're all prone to it.'[43]

A growing body of research reinforces Campbell's point.[42] We all have difficulties making certain complex judgements and decisions, and we resort to shortcuts when the mental strain becomes too great. Indeed, it is plausible to speculate that the reason why teacher assessment is biased is because it is so burdensome: when we are faced with difficult cognitive challenges, we often default to stereotypes. Exams are certainly unreliable due to variations in student performance on the day. However, it is by no means clear that this type of unreliability is worse than the systematic bias against disadvantaged pupils that results from teacher assessment.

In conclusion, descriptor-based models attempt to fulfil two different assessment purposes, but end up doing neither very well. They are unable to produce valid formative or summative information, and inconsistent summative grades are a particular problem for schools given that Ofsted scrutinise them in inspections. One obvious way to get more accurate grades is to use more formal exams, and in the next chapter we will look at assessment systems which are based on exams rather than descriptors.

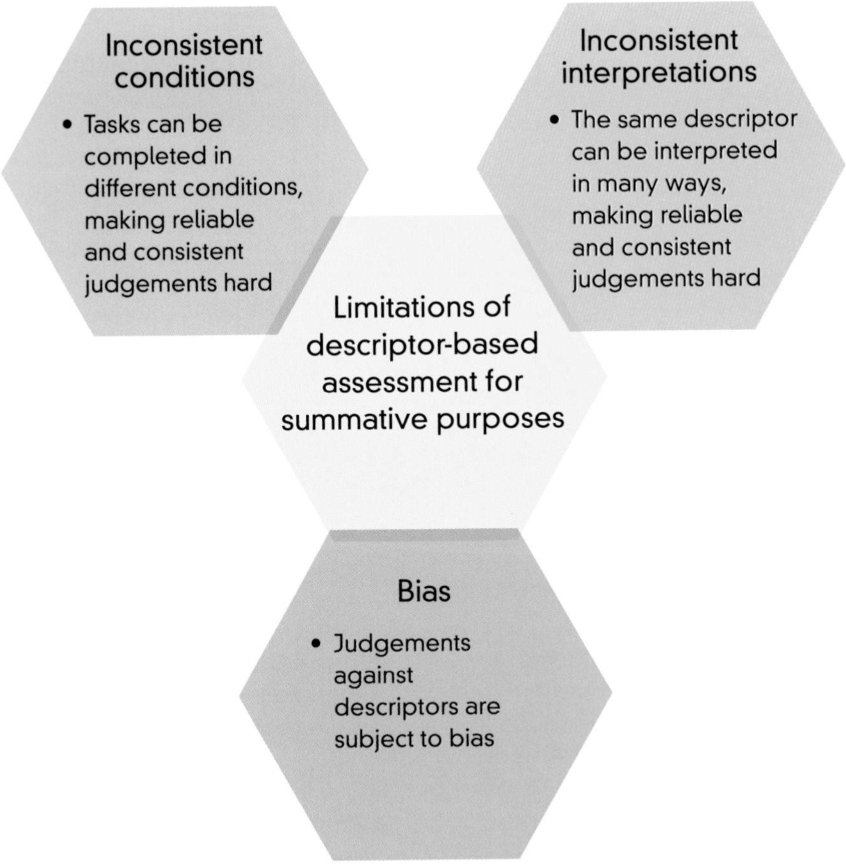

Inconsistent conditions

- Tasks can be completed in different conditions, making reliable and consistent judgements hard

Inconsistent interpretations

- The same descriptor can be interpreted in many ways, making reliable and consistent judgements hard

Limitations of descriptor-based assessment for summative purposes

Bias

- Judgements against descriptors are subject to bias

Figure 4.3: Limitations of descriptor-based assessment for summative purposes

Notes

1 Brill, F. and Twist, L, 2013. *Where Have All the Levels Gone? The Importance of a Shared Understanding of Assessment at a Time of Major Policy Change.* NFER Thinks: What the Evidence Tells Us. Slough: NFER, p.2

2 Department for Children, Schools and Families (known since 2010 as the Department for Education), 2009. *Getting to Grips with Assessing Pupils' Progress* <http://webarchive.nationalarchives.gov.uk/20130401151715/http://www.education.gov.uk/publications/eOrderingDownload/Assessing_pupils_progress.pdf> accessed 6 November 2016

3 The National Strategies. *Secondary: APP Writing* (archived) <http://webarchive.nationalarchives.gov.uk/20110809101133/http://wsassets.s3.amazonaws.com/ws/nso/pdf/44c1317f5bdb02732731cdf2820f45bb.pdf> accessed 6 November 2016

4 Department for Education, 2016. *Interim teacher assessment frameworks at the end of key stage 2* <https://www.gov.uk/government/publications/interim-frameworks-for-teacher-assessment-at-the-end-of-key-stage-2> accessed 6 November 2016

5 National Association of Head Teachers, 2014. *NAHT assessment framework materials* <http://www.naht.org.uk/welcome/news-and-media/key-topics/assessment/naht-assessment-framework-materials/?assetdeta8217081-91d4-4ed9-b39f-385fce55a32a=44636> accessed 6 November 2016

6 Pearson, 2016. *Pearson Progression Services: Progression Scale* <http://www.pearsonschoolsandfecolleges.co.uk/Secondary/Progression-Services/Progression-Services/Progression-Services/Progression-Scale/Progression-Scales.aspx> accessed 6 November 2016

7 Classroom Monitor, 2016. *Formative Assessment* <http://www.classroommonitor.co.uk/what-we-do/formative-assessment/> accessed 6 November 2016

8 Herts for Learning, 2015. *The Herts for Learning Approach to Tracking Pupil Progress (Primary)* <https://www.hertsforlearning.co.uk/sites/default/files/user_uploads/00_news/documents/hfl_approach_to_tracking_pupil_progress_dec2015.pdf> accessed 6 November 2016

9 EES for Schools, 2016. *Steps* <http://www.eesforschools.org/targettracker/steps> accessed 6 November 2016

10 EES for Schools, 2016. *Target Tracker* <http://www.eesforschools.org/targettracker> accessed 6 November 2016

11 Classroom Monitor, 2016. *Primary Schools* <http://www.classroommonitor.co.uk/school/pupil-tracking-primary-schools/> accessed 6 November 2016

12 Qualifications and Curriculum Development Agency, 2010. *The National Curriculum: level descriptions for subjects* <http://deraioe.ac.uk/10747/>; Department for Education. *Assessing Pupils' Progress (APP): Assessment guidelines* (archived) <http://webarchive.nationalarchives.gov.uk/20110809101133/nsonline.org.uk/node/20683>; Department for Education, 2016. *Interim teacher assessment frameworks at the end of key stage 2* <https://www.gov.uk/government/publications/interim-frameworks-for-teacher-assessment-at-the-end-of-key-stage-2>; National Association of Head Teachers, 2014. *NAHT assessment*

framework materials <http://www.naht.org.uk/welcome/news-and-media/key-topics/assessment/naht-assessment-framework-materials/?assetdeta8217081-91d4-4ed9-b39f-385fce55a32a=44636>; Herts for Learning, 2015. *HfL Assessment Criteria for Phase B Steps 4/5/6 (based on curriculum expectations for Year 4): Writing across a range of texts – Composition* <https://www.hertsforlearning.co.uk/sites/default/files/user_uploads/02_resources/documents/writing_assessment_criteria_y4_sample.pdf>; EES for Schools, 2016. *Target Tracker* <http://www.eesforschools.org/targettracker> all accessed 6 November 2016

13 Qualifications and Curriculum Development Agency, 2010. *Assessing pupils' progress: learners at the heart of assessment*, p.13 <https://www.essex.gov.uk/Business-Partners/Partners/Schools/One-to-one-tuition/Documents/Assessing%20Pupil%20Progress%20Learners%20at%20the%20heart%20of%20assessment.pdf> accessed 6 November 2016

14 Hertfordshire Grid for Learning, 2009. *Student Friendly APP Assessment Focuses* <http://thegrid.org.uk/learning/english/ks3-4-5/ks3/assessment/index.shtml#app> accessed 6 November 2016

15 Qualifications and Curriculum Development Agency, 2008. *Evaluation of the assessing pupils' progress in key stage 2 pilot project, 2006–2008*, pp.60–61 <http://archive.teachfind.com/qcda/www.qcda.gov.uk/resources/publication75b3.html?id=536c274d-1101-49b4-ba4f-b82ab7c8418b> accessed 6 November 2016

16 EES for Schools. *Steps User Guide* <http://www.eesforschools.org/TargetTracker/steps/Steps-User-Guide.pdf> accessed 6 November 2016

17 Classroom Monitor. *Pupil Tracking.* <http://www.classroommonitor.co.uk/what-we-do/pupil-tracking/> accessed 6 November 2016

18 Quoted in Wiliam, D. and Black, P., 1996. Meanings and Consequences: a basis for distinguishing formative and summative functions of assessment?. *British Educational Research Journal*, 22(5), pp.537–548

19 Department for Children, Schools and Families (known since 2010 as the Department for Education), 2008. *Assessing pupils' progress in English at Key Stage 3: Teachers' handbook*, p.17 <http://webarchive.nationalarchives.gov.uk/20130401151715/http://www.education.gov.uk/publications/eOrderingDownload/sec_eng_app_hndbk.pdf> accessed 6 November 2016

20 See, for example, McNamara, D. and Kintsch, W., 1996. Learning from texts: Effect of prior knowledge and text coherence. *Discourse Processes*, 22, pp.247–288

21 Laufer, B., 1996. The lexical plight in second language reading: Words you don't know, words you think you know, and words you can't guess. In Coady, J. and Huckin, T., eds. *Second Language Vocabulary Acquisition: A Rationale for Pedagogy*. Cambridge: Cambridge University Press, pp.20–34

22 Welsh Joint Education Committee (CBAC), 2006. *GCSE Examiners' Report Summer 2006: English & English Literature*, p.19 <http://www.kcse-online.info/gcse/uploads/publications/g-xr-english-s-06.pdf> accessed 4 March 2013

23 Beck, I.L, McKeown, M.G. and Kucan, L, 2013. *Bringing Words to Life: Robust Vocabulary Instruction* (second edition). New York: The Guilford Press, p.185

24 Department for Education, 2010. *The National Strategies: Assessing Pupils' Progress: A teachers' handbook*, p.5 <http://webarchive.nationalarchives. gov.uk/20110202093118/http:/nationalstrategies.standards.dcsf.gov.uk/ node/259613> accessed 6 November 2016

25 *Ibid.* p.22

26 British Columbia Ministry of Education, June 2004. *History 12 Resource A Exam Booklet*, p.8

27 Wiliam, D., 2011. *Embedded formative assessment*. Indiana: Solution Tree Press, pp.107–113

28 Soderstrom, N.C. and Bjork, R.A, 2013. Learning versus performance. In Dunn, D.S., ed. *Oxford bibliographies online: Psychology*. New York: Oxford University Press

29 Department for Children, Schools and Families (known since 2010 as the Department for Education). *The National Strategies: Assessing Pupils' Progress (APP) in mathematics: Criteria levels 1 to 8* <http://webarchive.nationalarchives. gov.uk/20110809101133/http://wsassets.s3.amazonaws.com/ws/nso/pdf/ ded0a20eb9380ce167ae919b000fe132.pdf> accessed 6 November 2016

30 Hart, K.M., quoted in Wiliam, D., 2014. *Principled Assessment Design*. London: SSAT: pp.65–66

31 Bambrick-Santoyo, P., 2010. *Driven by Data: A Practical Guide to Improve Instruction*. New Jersey: John Wiley & Sons, pp.6-7

32 Department for Children, Schools and Families (known since 2010 as the Department for Education). *The National Strategies: APP Reading: Assessment Focuses and Criteria* <http://webarchive.nationalarchives. gov.uk/20110809101133/http://wsassets.s3.amazonaws.com/ws/nso/ pdf/44c1317f5bdb02732731cdf2820f45bb.pdf> accessed 6 November 2016

33 Koretz, D., 1998. Large-scale Portfolio Assessments in the US: evidence pertaining to the quality of measurement. *Assessment in Education: Principles, Policy & Practice*, 5(3), pp.309–334

34 Wolf, A, 1998. Portfolio assessment as national policy: The National Council for Vocational Qualifications and its quest for a pedagogical revolution. *Assessment in Education: Principles, Policy & Practice*, 5(3), pp.413–445

35 Polanyi, M., 2012. *Personal Knowledge: Towards a Post-Critical Philosophy*. London: Routledge

36 Kuhn, T.S., 2012. *The Structure of Scientific Revolutions*. Chicago: University of Chicago Press

37 Bevan, R.M. et al., 2004. *A systematic review of the evidence of reliability and validity of assessment by teachers used for summative purposes*. London: EPPI-Centre, Social Science Research Unit, Institute of Education, University of London

38 Shorrocks, D., Daniels, S., Staintone, R and Ring, K, 1993. *Testing and Assessing 6 and 7 year olds: The Evaluation of the 1992 Key Stage 1 National Curriculum Assessment*. London: National Union of Teachers and Leeds University School of Education

39 Thomas, S., Madaus, G.F., Raczek, A.E. and Smees R, 1998. Comparing Teacher Assessment and the Standard Task Results in England: the relationship between pupil characteristics and attainment. *Assessment in Education: Principles, Policy & Practice*, 5, pp.213–246

40 Burgess, S. and Greaves, E., 2009. *Test Scores, Subjective Assessment and Stereotyping of Ethnic Minorities*. Bristol: Centre for Market and Public Organisation, University of Bristol

41 Campbell, T., 2015. Stereotyped at Seven? Biases in Teacher Judgement of Pupils' Ability and Attainment. *Journal of Social Policy*, 44(3), pp.517–547

42 Kahneman, D., 2011. *Thinking, Fast and Slow*. New York: Farrar, Straus and Giroux

43 Quoted in Adams, R, 2015. Children from poorer families perceived by teachers as less able, says study. *The Guardian*, 9 June <https://www.theguardian.com/education/2015/jun/09/teachers-poorer-children-education-primary-school> accessed 6 November 2016

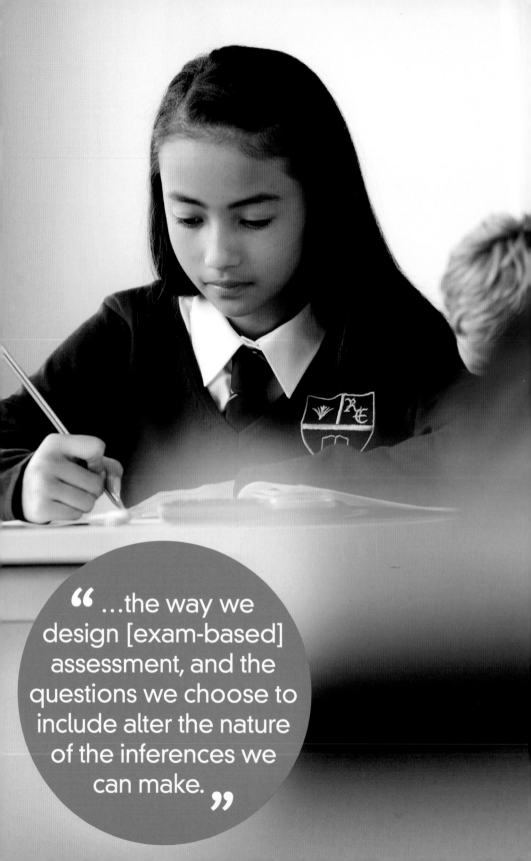

❝ …the way we design [exam-based] assessment, and the questions we choose to include alter the nature of the inferences we can make. **❞**

Exam-based assessment

5

How does this model work?

We saw in the previous chapter that descriptor-based assessment struggles to produce valid formative or summative information. One obvious way of getting more valid summative grades is to use formal tests, rather than aggregating classwork. In many cases, this was the system that existed before any descriptor-based models: one of the guides to APP noted that, before it was introduced, many schools used optional national test papers (commonly known as SATs) throughout the year to find out what level their pupils were working at.[1] In years 10 and 11, schools can use GCSE past papers to find out what grade their pupils are working at.

Whereas a descriptor-based model works by taking evidence from a range of classroom assessments, an exam-based model works by isolating the task that is to be used to make the summative inference. This means that the conditions can be more formal and standardised, as can the task itself. These tasks have been designed for summative purposes, but it is possible to analyse them with a formative purpose in mind. Wiliam and Black themselves suggested that 'the results of an assessment that had been designed originally to fulfil a summative function might be used formatively, as is the case when a teacher administers a paper from a previous year in order to help students to prepare for an examination.'[2]

In practice, therefore, a school could administer a past SATs or GCSE test paper three to six times a year and record the grades pupils got on each one. They could then use details of the pupils' performance on each test to provide formative information about how they needed to improve.

In Chapter 3, we looked at the difference between exams based on the difficulty model, which ask pupils to answer a series of questions of increasing difficulty, and those based on the quality model, which ask pupils to do one task and then require an examiner to judge the quality of their performance on that task. Exams based on the difficulty model produce a lot of information in addition to the final grade: it is possible to record not just the overall summative grade, but also each pupil's performance on each individual question. This approach, often called a question-level analysis or a gap analysis, allows teachers to see quickly which questions were particularly easy or difficult, as well as which pupils did particularly well or badly. This analysis could even be supplemented with data on how pupils nationally performed on each question. It is then also possible to label each question based on its topic, and to provide a breakdown of how pupils did on each topic:

Name	S 1	N 2	H 3a	H 3b	H 3c	M 4a	M 4b	C 5	S 6a	S 6b	P 7	S 8	N 9	C 10a	C 10b	P 11a	P 11b	C 12a	C 12b	P 13	S 14	P 15	C 16	N 17	C 18	P 19	P 20	N 21	N 22	Total
Keith White	1	0	1	0	1	0	1	0	1	0	1	0	1	0	1	0	1	0	1	0	1	0	1	0	1	0	1	0	0	14
Blake MacLeod	0	1	0	1	0	1	0	1	0	1	0	1	0	1	0	1	0	1	0	1	0	1	0	1	0	1	0	0	1	14
Stewart Marshall	1	1	1	1	0	1	0	1	0	1	0	1	0	1	0	1	0	1	0	1	1	1	1	1	1	1	1	1	1	20
Eric Morrison	0	1	0	1	0	1	0	1	0	1	0	1	0	1	0	1	0	1	0	1	0	1	0	1	0	1	0	0	1	14
Max Sutherland	1	1	1	0	1	0	1	0	1	0	1	0	1	0	1	0	1	0	1	0	1	1	1	1	1	1	1	1	1	20
Sebastian Hemmings	0	1	0	1	0	1	0	1	0	1	0	1	0	1	0	1	0	1	0	1	0	1	0	1	0	1	0	0	1	14
Sophie Scott	1	1	1	0	1	0	1	0	1	0	1	0	1	0	1	0	1	0	1	0	1	1	1	1	1	1	1	1	1	19
Faith Bond	0	1	0	1	0	1	0	1	0	1	0	1	0	1	0	1	0	1	0	1	0	1	0	1	0	1	0	0	1	14
Amy Johnston	0	1	0	1	0	1	0	1	0	1	0	1	0	1	1	1	1	1	1	1	1	1	1	1	1	1	0	1	0	17
Stephanie McDonald	0	1	0	1	0	1	0	1	0	1	0	1	0	1	0	1	0	1	0	1	0	1	0	1	0	1	0	0	1	14
Grace Stewart	0	1	0	1	0	1	1	1	1	1	1	1	0	1	0	1	0	1	0	1	1	1	1	1	1	1	1	1	1	23
Bernadette Newman	0	1	0	1	0	1	0	1	1	1	0	1	0	1	0	1	0	1	0	1	0	1	0	1	0	1	0	0	1	14
Deirdre Harris	1	0	1	0	1	1	1	1	1	1	1	1	0	1	0	1	0	1	1	1	1	1	1	1	1	1	1	1	1	23
Joseph Skinner	0	1	0	1	0	1	0	1	0	1	0	1	0	1	0	1	0	1	0	1	0	1	0	1	0	1	0	0	1	14
Bella Taylor	0	1	0	1	0	1	1	1	1	1	1	1	0	1	0	1	0	1	0	1	1	1	1	1	1	1	1	0	1	22
Lillian Graham	0	1	0	1	0	1	0	1	0	1	0	1	0	1	0	1	0	1	0	1	0	1	0	1	0	1	0	0	1	14
Ruth Nolan	0	1	0	1	0	1	0	1	0	1	0	1	0	1	0	1	0	1	0	1	0	1	1	1	1	1	1	1	1	17
Felicity Clark	0	1	0	1	1	1	0	1	0	1	0	1	0	1	0	1	0	1	0	1	0	1	0	1	0	1	0	0	1	15
Zoe Nolan	0	1	0	1	1	1	0	1	0	1	0	1	0	1	0	1	0	1	0	1	0	1	0	1	0	1	0	0	1	15
Elizabeth Churchill	0	1	0	1	1	1	0	1	0	1	0	1	0	1	0	1	0	1	0	1	0	1	0	1	0	1	0	0	1	15
Donna Blake	0	1	0	1	1	1	0	1	0	1	0	1	0	1	0	1	0	1	0	0	0	0	0	0	0	0	0	0	1	12
Connor Hodges	0	1	0	1	1	1	0	1	0	1	0	1	0	1	0	1	0	1	0	1	0	1	0	1	0	1	0	0	1	15
Gordon Bailey	0	1	0	1	1	1	0	1	0	1	0	1	0	1	0	1	0	1	0	1	0	1	1	1	1	1	1	0	1	17
Alison Mitchell	0	1	0	1	1	1	0	1	0	1	0	1	0	1	0	1	0	1	0	1	0	1	1	1	1	1	1	0	1	18
Wanda Randall	0	1	0	1	1	1	0	1	0	1	0	1	0	1	0	1	0	1	0	1	0	1	0	1	0	1	0	0	1	15
Stephanie Baker	0	1	0	1	1	1	0	1	0	1	0	1	0	1	0	1	0	1	0	1	0	1	0	1	0	1	0	0	1	15
Thomas Walsh	0	1	0	1	1	1	0	0	0	0	0	0	0	0	0	0	0	1	0	1	0	1	0	1	0	1	0	0	1	10
Felicity Robertson	0	1	0	1	0	1	0	1	0	1	0	1	0	1	0	1	0	1	1	1	1	1	1	1	1	1	1	1	1	19
Harry Berry	0	1	0	1	0	1	0	1	0	1	0	1	0	1	0	1	0	1	0	1	0	1	0	1	0	1	0	0	1	14
Faith North	0	1	0	1	0	1	0	1	0	1	0	1	0	1	0	1	0	1	0	1	0	1	0	1	0	1	0	0	1	14
% Correct	17%	93%	17%	87%	50%	87%	23%	35%	37%	70%	37%	70%	33%	63%	33%	63%	37%	63%	43%	70%	47%	80%	48%	85%	45%	85%	48%	20%		

Figure 5.1: Question-level analysis spreadsheet

for example, one could look not just at a pupil's performance in maths but at the breakdown of results in number, shape and data handling topics. Based on this, a teacher would be able to work out which areas his or her teaching should focus on next. Figure 5.1 shows a question-level analysis spreadsheet for a maths exam which uses the difficulty model.[3]

This spreadsheet is taken from the Times Educational Supplement (TES) resources website, and has been filled in with fake pupil data. It was designed to be used with the 2014 Maths SATs paper. In the first column are the names of all the pupils in a class. Each successive column records whether they got a particular question right or wrong. This allows each pupil's score to be aggregated in the final column. It also allows the teacher to see what percentage of pupils got each question right by looking at the bottom row. In this case, the spreadsheet has been colour coded to show questions that a high percentage of pupils have got right, as well as wrong. In this example, 70% of pupils got question 13 correct, so the spreadsheet formula has automatically highlighted this cell green. Only 17% got question 1 right, so the spreadsheet has automatically highlighted this cell red. In row 3, each question has also been categorised as one of six different topics: shape and space (S), handling data (H), measurement (M), calculation (C), problem solving (P) and number (N). One can then click on the other tabs in the spreadsheet to see a breakdown of the scores by topic.

This spreadsheet has been designed for use with primary SATs tests, but such approaches might be even more common at GCSE level. PiXL, the school improvement organisation, which approximately 1,500 secondary schools in England belonged to as of September 2016, developed a maths app based on similar principles. Pupils can take a past exam paper, and the app calculates their areas of strength and weakness based on the questions they got right and wrong.[4]

When exams are based on the quality model, question-level analysis is a little trickier. A maths paper might have 50 or 60 questions, but an English or history paper might only have four or five. In principle, the same question-level analysis is possible, but each of those four or five questions will require some marker judgement in a way that the maths or science questions will not. This judgement will probably be supported by a rubric or prose descriptors and, when it is, we face the same problems with descriptors we saw in the previous chapter. Therefore, in some subjects, what looks like an exam-based assessment model still relies to a large extent on descriptors.

Does the exam-based model provide valid formative information?

Although this model was not designed with formative inferences in mind, question-level analysis clearly does allow for such inferences to be made. How valid are they? In some ways, the information from these analyses is very useful. Some of the questions they are based on are quite specific, so knowing if a pupil got a particular question right or wrong allows the teacher to provide specific feedback. Indeed, one of the major figures in the development of standardised tests in the US, E.F. Lindquist, argued that the questions on such tests should be as specific as possible in order to allow for useful feedback. Koretz summarises this school of thought as follows:

> If one breaks skills and knowledge into small pieces, one can more easily ascertain which specific skills contribute to students' weaknesses and thus help educators improve their teaching. For example, if we can pinpoint the specific missing skills that cause students to perform poorly on problems with fractions, a teacher or school administrator may be able to improve the teaching of those particular skills.
>
> Koretz, D., *Measuring Up*, p.49

Koretz also gives more information about how this approach would work in practice:

> *To help guide instruction, Lindquist wanted as much as practical*
> *to isolate specific knowledge and skills. In his view, this required*
> *designing tests to include tasks that focus narrowly on these specifics.*
> *For example, Lindquist would have argued that if you want to*
> *determine whether third-grade students can manage subtraction*
> *with carrying, you give them problems that require subtraction with*
> *carrying but that entail as few ancillary skills as possible. You would*
> *not embed that skill in complex text, because then a student might*
> *fail to solve the problem either for want of these arithmetic skills or*
> *because of poor reading, and it would be hard to know which.*
>
> Koretz, D., *Measuring Up*, pp.42–43

There are plenty of questions in summative tests which are as specific as this, and which give the teacher useful feedback about their teaching, whole-class performance and the performance of individuals. For example, question 16 on the 2014 maths SATs paper was 'Calculate 465×52'.[5] Pupils who got that question wrong may need some practice with multiplying two- and three-digit numbers. If the whole class got it wrong, the teacher may look back at the lessons he taught on that skill and look to see if there was anything he could improve. If the whole class got it right, the teacher might want to share his lesson plans for this topic with his colleagues.

Supplementing these spreadsheets with data on national performance can make them even more useful. For example, knowing the percentage of pupils nationally who correctly answered '465×52' adds some important context. Suppose 25% of pupils in a class got that question right. A teacher's decision about what to do next in class might be affected by the national success rate. If 75% of pupils nationally got that question right, a teacher might decide to focus on reteaching that skill. However, if only 10% nationally got the question right, the teacher might decide there are more pressing priorities. Even if national data is not available, comparing data within a school can yield useful formative insights. If two classes with similar ability profiles had very different success rates for a question, then the two teachers could share notes and see what they had done differently. Perhaps, in one class a pupil asked a question that helped to clear up a common misconception, or one teacher added in a step that was particularly helpful.

Whilst this is an example of how exams can be used to give useful feedback, unfortunately not all questions are, or can be, this precise. We saw in Chapter 3 that summative exams need to sample from a large domain, have questions that distinguish between candidates, and be taken in standard conditions. The first two of these are reasons why questions taken from summative exams cannot be as precise and specific as they would be if they had been designed first and foremost with formative inferences in mind. As a result, they cannot all provide as useful formative information as the example we've just looked at. A third factor also reduces the value of the formative information from this system, which is that this system measures all progress through improvements in summative grades or sub-grades. However, summative grades are not sensitive enough to measure formative progress, which means that genuine progress goes unrecorded, and superficial and shallow progress is rewarded instead.

Tests are samples from a domain, not direct measurements

First, summative exams are samples of a domain, not direct measurements. Let's briefly recap what it means for an exam to be a sample. Exams do not directly measure everything a pupil knows. Instead, they take a small sample and use that to make an inference about the knowledge in the wider domain. That's fine for an inference about maths, for example, but it is not fine for an inference about the subcategories that make up a maths exam. A typical maths exam might have 50 or 60 questions; the 2014 SATs paper featured at the start of this chapter has 65. Those 65 maths questions can provide a reliable inference about a pupil's maths ability. However, when we look at the different topics this maths exam covers, we can see that there are only about 5–15 questions on each of the different areas. There are only 7 questions on data handling, for example. As a result, it simply isn't possible to make reliable inferences about all the subcategories we are interested in from one summative exam.[6] The only way around this is to make the test longer.[7] The more questions that are included in a test, the less the sampling unreliability. The problem with this, of course, is that to get a test that did give reliable scores on all these subcategories, we would need one with hundreds of questions that would take hours, perhaps even days, to answer. If we want to make an inference about whether we need to spend more time on a particular subtopic, then exam analysis cannot provide us with that answer. Nor can such analysis allow us to measure progress on subtopics over time. We do not have enough evidence from one summative maths exam to make an inference about, for example, a pupil's attainment in data handling. If we then try to look at two different summative exams from different points in time and measure the progress a pupil has made in data handling between the two, we are just multiplying error.

Questions on tests range in difficulty

Second, questions in summative exams range in difficulty so that they can distinguish between candidates. More difficult questions combine different topics, which makes it hard to know exactly why a pupil might have got the question wrong. If all that is recorded on the question-level analysis is whether a pupil got the mark for the question or not, it is impossible to work out why they got it wrong. Take the following science exam question:

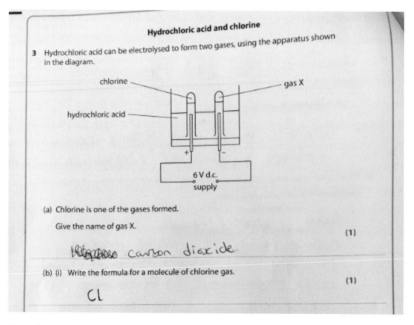

Figure 5.2: Science GCSE exam question as featured on thescienceteacher.co.uk

On the surface, this is a question about electrolysis, but we can see from the pupil response to this question that this pupil is struggling not with the principles of electrolysis but with far more fundamental issues. One science teacher who has analysed this paper describes it as follows:

Let's look at 3(a). The student gets this answer wrong. But more interesting than that, the student states it was carbon dioxide and therefore demonstrates a more fundamental misunderstanding, they don't know that elements are always conserved in chemical reactions. The only possible substances that could be formed from HCl are hydrogen or chlorine. If they did understand this concept of conservation, then carbon dioxide could never have been an option. It is possible they think carbon dioxide contains H or Cl atoms but whatever the 'gap', I don't think it will be addressed with revision of electrolysis.

Now let's look at 3(b). The student states that the formula of a molecule of chlorine is Cl instead of Cl_2. The student clearly does not understand the concept of diatomic molecules. Simply reviewing the paper in class and getting students to make corrections will only bring about progress if that exact question appears again. A much more effective approach would be to review diatomic molecules and covalent bonding as this is not a misunderstanding of electrolysis per se.

Green, J., Question level analysis in science

In this case, careful analysis of the exam question could provide useful feedback, but this more nuanced information is not captured in a question-level spreadsheet: all that is recorded is whether the pupil got the question right or wrong. And whilst on this occasion we were able to work out what the problem really was, there are many occasions where even careful analysis of responses will not help. For example, suppose a 12-year-old pupil is struggling to read because they are not yet a fluent decoder of text. Their performance on an unseen comprehension exam will also be impeded by the fact that they are a poor decoder of text. However, it will be hard to infer reliably from their answers that this is the case. The errors they make might look the same as pupils who are good decoders but who have a poor vocabulary. To establish the exact reason for their poor performance, you would need some kind of phonics test. This would help identify some useful next steps for the pupils who struggled on this test. However, this test would not be particularly useful summatively, because most 12-year-olds would get full marks on it.

Something similar is true in maths. Some pupils will fail to answer a question about the area of a rectangle because they don't understand how to calculate the area of a rectangle. Others will struggle because their knowledge of basic number facts and times tables is weak. Even if pupils show their working, it is hard to infer reliably exactly what the source of their struggles is, and it is even harder to record such information on a question-level analysis spreadsheet.

If one combined the phonics questions and the comprehension questions, or the times tables grids and the complex questions on algebra, then it would be possible to get a test which offered reliable formative information about every pupil, as well as a valid summative grade. The problem, again, would be that to do this one would need tests that were prohibitively long. Such tests would also require some pupils spending hours answering questions that were far too hard for them, and others answering lots of questions that were far too easy.

The more difficult – and indeed the more authentic – the question, the more likely it is that a pupil will fail for reasons that have nothing to do with their skill in that subject. Earlier, we saw Koretz summarise the argument against authentic questions: when assessing a skill, 'you would not embed that skill in complex text, because then a student might fail to solve the problem either for want of these arithmetic skills or because of poor reading, and it would be hard to know which.'[8] But we know that many, many questions in summative exams are embedded in complex text. For example, the following maths question is, on the surface, about measurement and might be coded as such in a question-level analysis spreadsheet:[9]

Margaret is in Switzerland.
The local supermarket sells boxes
of Reblochon cheese.

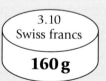

Each box of Reblochon cheese costs 3.10 Swiss francs.
It weighs 160 g.
In England, a box of Reblochon cheese costs £13.55 per kg.
The exchange rate is £1 = 1.65 Swiss francs.
Work out whether Reblochon cheese is better value for money in Switzerland or in England.

Plenty of pupils could have a good understanding of measurement, but struggle to answer such a question because they were unaware of what Reblochon is or what Swiss francs are. We might think that details like these are easy to ignore, but in practice they can confuse and distract pupils, particularly pupils with weak reading skills.

As a side note, one can argue about whether such questions do indeed allow us to make the summative inferences we are interested in. Different users of exam information might have different ideas about this. The manager of a chain of grocery stores might like such questions, as they allow her to make a good inference about who is suited to work in her store. The admissions tutor at a further education college might not like such questions, as they do not allow him to make a good inference about which pupils could flourish on a maths A level, given a little tuition in English. Koretz makes a similar argument about inferences. He imagines taking a maths exam in Hebrew, a language which he cannot speak or read well, and asks:

> What should the admissions officers have concluded about me based on my dismal score? If they had concluded that I lacked the mathematical and other cognitive abilities needed for university study, they would have been wrong...Now suppose they wanted to answer the question: whether I was at that time and with the proficiency I had then, likely to be successful in Hebrew language university study? In that case my low score would have been right on the money: I would have been a weak student indeed.
>
> Koretz, D., *Measuring Up*, p.310

The very same assessment can be used to produce two very different inferences. Moreover, the way we design that assessment – and the questions we choose to include – alters the nature of the inferences we can make. If we decide to include more complex and authentic tasks in maths papers, it is likely that pupils with better literacy skills will get better scores. This may be acceptable given that some of the inferences people want to make will involve a pupil's ability to do such real-world maths problems.

Whilst there is clearly a case for and against such tasks being used in summative exams, their formative value is much less clear. Such tasks are not designed for diagnosing why pupils are struggling. There are different and very distinctive ways in which a pupil might fail at the Reblochon cheese question; those ways are not apparent at all from a binary record of whether they got the question right or not, or even from analysis of their workings.

Question-level analysis is a powerful tool, but its value depends on the nature of the questions that are being analysed. When such questions have been chosen with formative purposes in mind, then analysis of them is very useful, and we will look in more detail at this in Chapter 7. But in the exam-based model, the questions are from exams that have been designed with summative purposes in mind, and in these cases, question-level analysis leads to many of the problems we saw with the descriptor-based model. Just as the descriptor model is based on performance, not learning, so too exam questions are selected according to grading principles, not learning principles.

This problem is even more acute in those subjects, like English, which follow a quality model of assessment. In these exams, there are none of the easy-to-interpret, specific questions that we looked at earlier and, instead, pupils are often given just one or two lengthy and complex tasks where it is difficult to infer the causes of success or failure. For example, a pupil might be given a reading passage and asked to answer four questions on it. Suppose the first question is a search-and-retrieve question which asks pupils to find certain pieces of information in a section of the text. If a pupil performs poorly on such a question, then the formative inference that seems most obvious is that they are poor at search-and-retrieve questions and need more practice on these types of question. But again, this inference is based on a pupil's understanding of just a few sentences of text. If there are just a few words in those sentences that a pupil does not understand, that will be enough for them to perform poorly on that question. We don't have enough information from this one question on a few lines of text to infer with enough certainty that the pupil has a problem with searching and retrieving text.

Examiners' reports show how difficult it is to interpret such answers in a formative way. These reports are written by the chief examiner and offer some qualitative information about how pupils performed on particular national exams. In plenty of these reports, the chief examiners themselves concede that they are not able to work out exactly why pupils struggled with certain questions, and this is particularly the case with reading exams. For example, one GCSE reading test featured a newspaper article on the Grand National, which pupils struggled with for reasons which were not clear to the examiner:

I thought that I might be apologising for how embarrassingly straightforward this question was but it proved to be inexplicably difficult as many of the candidates just could not focus their minds on the reasons why the Grand National is such a dangerous race. I know that comparison has always been difficult but this question was set up to make things as straightforward as possible. Still it seemed like an insurmountable hurdle, the examining equivalent of Becher's Brook, at which large numbers fell dramatically. I cannot really explain why so many candidates got themselves into such a tangle with this question. Many of them went round in circles, asserting that the race was dangerous because it was dangerous.

WJEC, *GSCE Examiners' Reports English and English Language*, p.12

These responses are perhaps not as inexplicable as the examiner suggests. The problem the examiner identifies about circular reasoning – 'the race was dangerous because it was dangerous' – is one that pupils often resort to when they know they have to try and give a reason, but they don't know what the reason is. We saw exactly this in the first chapter, where Willingham said: 'if you remind a student to "look at an issue from multiple perspectives" often enough, he will learn that he ought to do so, but if he doesn't know much about an issue, he *can't* think about it from multiple perspectives.'[10] We can perhaps infer from this common response that these pupils had been well-prepared on exam technique, and clearly knew they had to give a reason why the race was dangerous. However, they did not understand the text well enough to be able to offer a reason, and the reason why they did not understand the text was due to the unfamiliar subject matter and perhaps also some difficult vocabulary. The best next step, therefore, would be to set up a structured programme that aimed to develop vocabulary and background knowledge. Still, even though we have attempted an explanation and a suggestion of feedback here, the examiner is right to note that there is still a lot we cannot explain, and any feedback will lack specificity because we just don't have the information we need to produce something more specific.

Another examiner's report shows something similar:

Most candidates were able to gain a mark for the next part of the question stating that the whale shark eats plankton. However a number of candidates offered no answer, perhaps they did not recognise plankton to be food, although the context should have made this clear.
WJEC, *GCSE Examiners' Reports English, English Language and English Literature,* p.4

Why did a number of candidates offer no answer? Again, we cannot be certain. Was it because they had never come across the word plankton before? Later on, the examiner suggests that the problem may have been that 'they failed to read the article properly.' Again, it is hard to know with any certainty; there are a few plausible reasons, and it is hard to work out what the best feedback or next steps would be for the pupil.

A third examiner's report shows how writing tasks require a complex set of knowledge and skills, as well as how pupils might struggle with such tasks because of aspects that are not a part of any writing curriculum:

> *Although candidates were able, on the whole, to give a cogent account of life in the city, the perceptions of life 'on a small island' were less clear and less persuasive in pursuance of their argument. Despite the work they had already done on Source 2 – which featured a small island, and from which the impetus for the question arose – there were some esoteric notions of what life would be like in such a place, ranging from it being a place of extreme heat, palm trees and sand, to a place devoid of jobs, communication, education and even food, where one would be severed from friends and family.*
>
> AQA, GCSE English/English Language: Report on the Examination, p.4

This is particularly interesting because it acknowledges that a lack of knowledge about a topic – in this case, what life is like on an island – has an impact on the clarity and persuasiveness of a pupil's writing. That is, within one exam paper, a pupil's ability to write clearly and persuasively differs based on the presence or absence of background knowledge. Still, whilst this report does suggest a reason why pupils struggled at a particular question, again, it is not straightforward to make this diagnosis, and it is not easy to create specific feedback in response to it either. In short, summative exams have to include complex tasks, but the more complex the task, the less useful it is formatively.

Grades aren't designed to measure formative progress

The third reason why this model fails to provide useful formative information is that it measures all progress through improvement in summative grades. In theory, one of the strengths of this model is that by isolating the task designed to produce summative information, it frees up the rest of the teaching time to be used for more flexible and responsive tasks. However, in practice, this system measures progress through the improvements in grades on summative tests. This ends up exerting just as much pressure on the curriculum as the descriptor-based model.

For example, imagine a maths teacher who has spent a term teaching pupils about fractions. At the end of the term, the pupils take a summative SATs or GCSE exam paper and the teacher compares their grade on that assessment with their grade from their most recent assessment, the term before, which was also a summative exam paper. Most of the questions on these exam papers will not be about fractions, so measuring progress from paper to paper by looking at the overall improvement in grade will not give a reliable measure of the progress pupils have made on fractions.

As we've seen, even if one were to isolate the questions on fractions and just look at those, that would not give a reliable measure of progress on fractions either. It is therefore entirely possible for a pupil to have studied fractions for a term, made significant progress in their understanding of fractions, and for their overall grade on a summative exam to either stay the same or get worse. If this is the only piece of data that is recorded and communicated with pupils, it is very misleading. This method of assessment might be a way of measuring summative progress against very big domains, but it is precisely because they measure such large domains that they are blunt and insensitive instruments when it comes to measuring progress over smaller domains and spans of time.

The problem is that this incentivises superficial teaching approaches. Why study fractions or sentence structures when there is such a small chance that progress on these domains will show up on the end-of-unit assessment? It is very hard to make genuine and significant improvements on such big domains over just six weeks. Valuable activities which will pay dividends in the long term will not show up on these assessments in the short term.

The risk is that if teachers are held accountable to short-term progress on these assessments, they will end up prioritising activities which don't lead to significant long-term learning but which do lead to quick, yet misleading, short-term gains.

Instead of spending time developing pupils' understanding of sentence structure, the temptation will be to get them to memorise a couple of impressive introductory sentences for the essay that will be used as the end-of-unit assessment. Instead of ensuring that pupils are completely fluent with their times tables, there will be a temptation to get them to develop a surface understanding of a new topic such as data handling. Although the first of each of these pairs of activities will lead to long-term learning, these real improvements will not show up on an exam-based assessment model. The second of each pair of activities do not lead to long-term learning, but they will lead to superficial improvements. Measuring progress with grades therefore encourages teaching to the test, which compromises learning. In the next chapter, we will look in more detail at teaching to the test and the problems it causes.

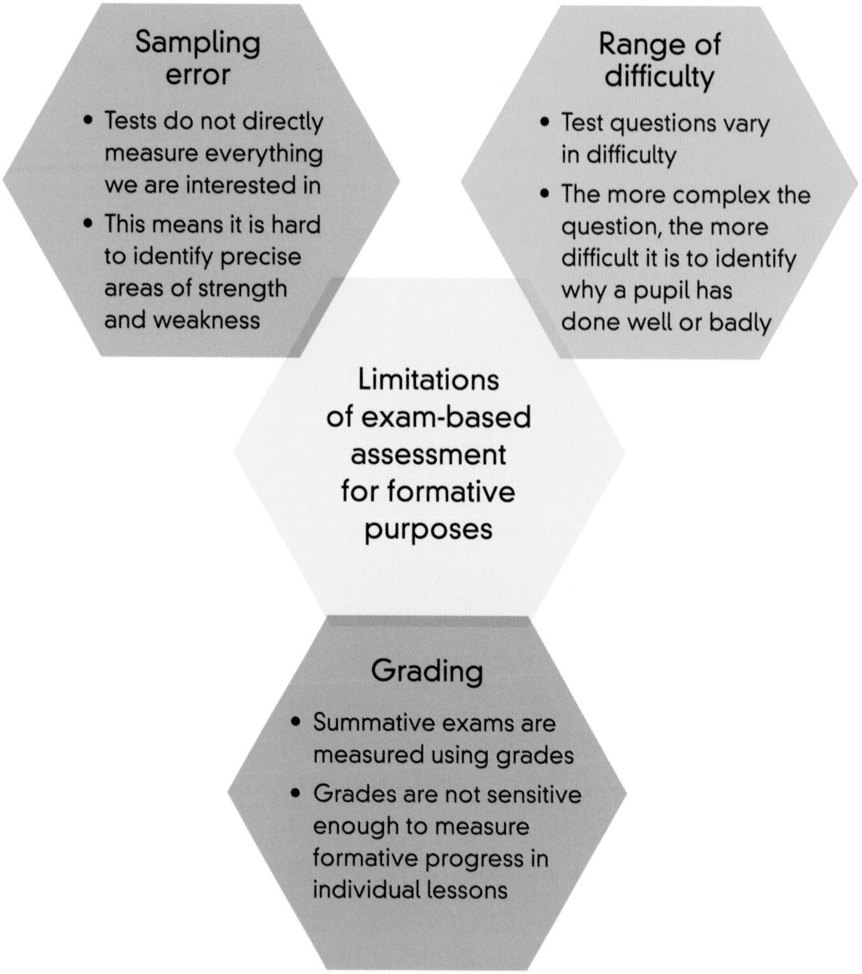

Sampling error

- Tests do not directly measure everything we are interested in
- This means it is hard to identify precise areas of strength and weakness

Range of difficulty

- Test questions vary in difficulty
- The more complex the question, the more difficult it is to identify why a pupil has done well or badly

Limitations of exam-based assessment for formative purposes

Grading

- Summative exams are measured using grades
- Grades are not sensitive enough to measure formative progress in individual lessons

Figure 5.3: Limitations of exam-based assessment for formative purposes

Does the exam-based model provide valid summative information?

The exam-based model has been designed to produce valid summative information and, in general, it does, but only if the exams being used are designed to produce such information. In practice, using exams that have been designed in this way imposes such restrictions that it is actually quite hard to stick to the routine of doing so, particularly when, as we have seen, the same tests are also expected to provide formative information. In order to see why this is, let's explore some of the restrictions imposed by summative tests in more detail.

In Chapter 3, we saw that in order to make a valid summative inference, exams must be taken in standardised conditions, sample from a wider domain and include questions of moderate difficulty that distinguish between pupils. As well as this, the results from such exams need to be reported using a consistent and comparable scale. This can actually be quite difficult to do, so it is worth further exploration.

We have seen that a simple statement or criterion such as 'can compare fractions to see which is larger' is capable of being interpreted in many different ways. It can be interpreted in such a way that many pupils will find quite simple to answer, for example, 'Which is bigger, $\frac{5}{7}$ or $\frac{3}{7}$?'. Or, it can be interpreted in such a way that many pupils will find quite tricky, for example, 'Which is bigger, $\frac{5}{7}$ or $\frac{5}{9}$?'. It is impossible to create a form of words that will allow people to define tasks with no ambiguity at all; there will always be room for different interpretations. Not only that, but it is also extremely hard for exam-setters – and indeed humans in general – to predict in advance the relative difficulty of different questions. We cannot say in advance just how difficult a group of pupils will find a question like 'Find $\frac{2}{5}$ of 35' compared with a question like 'Find $\frac{7}{8}$ of 56'. Similarly, if we have two unseen texts, we cannot say in advance how difficult one group will find one text compared to another.

This has huge implications for the setting of standards, grade boundaries and pass marks. It might seem obvious that we should say that, for example, on a maths exam a raw mark of between 60 and 69 should always correspond to a 'B' or to a standard of 'expected'. However, we are unable to say that, because different selections of questions will not be equally difficult. The problem becomes particularly acute when trying to set standards for different versions of the same exam. A 2014 version of an exam has to produce results that are consistent with the 2013 and 2015 versions, but it also has to feature different questions. Examiners need to select questions of comparable difficulty to the year before, but we know that even slight changes to a question can significantly affect how difficult pupils find it.[11] The best way of producing consistently difficult exams would be to have exactly the same exam from year to year. Of course, this would not actually then be consistently difficult because the pupils taking it in the second year would know exactly what questions to expect. So, the questions have to change, but in changing them we inevitably also change the difficulty of the exam.

One way around this problem of setting and maintaining standards is to use information about how difficult pupils found different questions. GL Assessment describe the process they use for developing tests:

> *Any standardised test will go through rigorous development and take*
> *between two and four years to complete. The test structure has to*
> *be modelled, a large amount of test content must be developed and*
> *trialled with students in schools and then refined through a statistical*
> *process to produce the final tests. These are standardised on a very*
> *large, representative sample of students usually across the UK.*
>
> GL Assessment, *A Short Guide to Standardised Tests*, p.3

Ultimately, this is the reason why grade boundaries fluctuate from exam to exam. Different exams have different questions in them and those different questions will have varying levels of difficulty. It isn't possible to predict in advance the relative difficulty of different questions, so a raw mark of 65 on one paper might represent the same standard as a 69 on another paper, or vice versa.[12]

This leads to a couple of implications for classroom practice. First of all, it means that using raw marks as a guide to making summative inferences is flawed. It can be tempting to use raw marks in this way, because they hold out the promise of finer distinctions than grades. However, raw marks obtained on different tests are not comparable.

Second, the difficulty of maintaining standards from test to test shows that it is extremely hard for any individual, or even school, to create tests with consistent standards. National exam boards and assessment organisations spend significant amounts of time and money trialling questions and moderating tasks in order to ensure that the grades they award are consistent over time. We can see, therefore, that not only are summative assessments restricted in terms of their structure, but that such restrictions make it hard for teachers to design them.

A system based around such tests would certainly provide valid summative information. However, given all the restrictions that such a system requires, it would be hard for teachers and schools to stick to it. This is particularly the case when such tests are also expected to provide formative information.

In practice, what often happens is that such tests are pulled between two purposes. Often, this can represent itself as a tension within schools between senior managers, who are often more concerned with accurate summative data, and teachers, who are often more concerned with useful formative data. Take the example we looked at earlier in this chapter, involving a unit on fractions, followed by a past GCSE paper. In this situation, a teacher might want to adapt the past paper so that it only includes questions on fractions as well as adapt the grade boundaries accordingly. They might argue that this would be a fairer representation of what the pupils have studied that term, and that the questions will also provide more useful feedback to pupils. A senior manager might query the grade derived from such a truncated paper on the grounds that it isn't accurate.

In a sense, both are right and both are wrong. The teacher is right to say that the most useful teaching tool is a test solely on fractions, but wrong to say that you can get the kind of summative grade required from a test that is solely on fractions. The senior manager is right to say that the test solely on fractions isn't giving a fair grade, but may be wrong to have requested such a grade in the first place. The real risk in such a situation is that schools end up using tests that fulfil neither function well: they have been adapted too much to give an accurate summative inference, but haven't been adapted enough to give the kind of focused feedback that is most valuable formatively.

There are other ways of adapting this system to fulfil both summative and formative purposes. For example, we could make the system more modular: instead of taking an exam every term which features a large spread of content, pupils can sit an exam, in standard conditions, which features a more concentrated focus on a smaller subcategory. At the end of the year, once pupils have taken five or six such exams, the teacher can then aggregate the scores from across these six exams. Although each exam on its own does not provide the spread of content needed for a summative inference, taken together, the six exams do. Indeed, in many ways, this could seem even better than a traditional end-of-year summative exam because, as the assessments can be split up over the year, it is possible to sample a much larger part of the overall subject domain. Instead of pupils taking a single two-hour maths exam at the end of the year, their maths grade can be based on six two-hour exams across the year.

This modular approach promises to offer the best of both worlds: summative inferences that are more accurate because they are based on a larger sample, and formative inferences that are more accurate because they can be closely linked to the specific work pupils are doing in class at a particular moment. In practice, however, this system also falls between two stools. Summative inferences need to be able to tell us something, not just about what a pupil can do at a particular moment in time, but about what they have truly learnt and what has changed in long-term memory.

One of the biggest threats to this inference is cramming, or, to give its technical term, massed practice. This is when pupils rely on intense, one-off, short-term study sessions. Such revision is effective at improving performance in the short-term but it is less effective at improving learning, so it is a threat to the kind of long-term summative inferences we want to make.[13–14] Cramming is a threat to terminal exams too, but it is more of a threat to modular exams because less content is covered in modular exams and so it is easier to cram for them. For example, if a pupil knows that the only time they will be tested on their understanding of *Great Expectations* is in an exam straight after they have finished studying it, and if there is nothing else on that exam but questions on *Great Expectations*, then the incentive is to cram their study of the novel into the period just before the exam and to neglect it afterwards. And indeed, when national exam systems have been based on modules, this is what has happened. After the introduction of A-level modules in 2000, one review noted that individual modules came to be seen almost as separate subjects, whilst another said that modules had led to 'compartmentalised learning' and made it harder for students to 'connect discrete areas of knowledge.'[15–16] When such systems are used for schools' internal assessment systems, Wiliam has noted the following:

> This results in what I call a 'banking' model of assessment in which once a student has earned a grade for an assignment, they get to keep that grade even if they subsequently forget everything they knew about this topic. It thus encourages a shallow approach to learning, and teaching. Students know that they only have to remember the material for two or three weeks until they take the test on that material, and they can then forget it, so there is no incentive for the student to gain the deep understanding that is needed for long-term recall.
>
> Wiliam, D., *What assessment can—and cannot—do*

Neither do these types of exam allow for very useful formative inferences to be made: the fact that the scores from them will eventually contribute towards a summative inference restricts their style and content in many of the ways we have discussed previously. Far from offering the best of both worlds, such systems actually offer the worst of both worlds: they significantly compromise the flexibility and responsiveness of formative assessments in order to be able to make a very uncertain summative inference.

Whilst the exam-based model might offer some improvements on the descriptors we saw in the previous chapter, in practice, both models have many similar flaws: they both expect the same assessment to provide formative and summative inferences, and as a result they both lead to over-frequent grading. In the final four chapters, we will look at some alternative systems which are based on different assumptions about assessment, learning and progress.

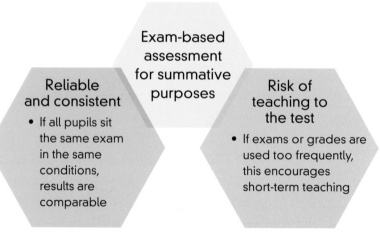

Figure 5.4: Exam-based assessment for summative purposes: strengths and risks

Notes

1 Department for Education, 2010. *The National Strategies: Assessing Pupils' Progress: A teachers' handbook*, pp.4-5

2 Wiliam, D. and Black, P., 1996. Meanings and Consequences: a basis for distinguishing formative and summative functions of assessment?, *British Educational Research Journal*, 22(5), pp.537–548

3 Urry, P. (eric_t_viking), 2014. *2014 detailed SATs question level analysis* <https://www.tes.com/teaching-resource/2014-detailed-sats-question-level-analysis-6437326> accessed 6 November 2016

4 The PiXL Club, 2016. *PiXL Maths App* <http://mathsapp.pixl.org.uk> accessed 6 November 2016

5 Standards and Testing Agency, 2014, *Mathematics tests, Key Stage 2, paper 1* <http://www.satspapers.org.uk/SATs_Papers/KS2_Maths/SATS_MATHS_2014%20KS2/2014_KS2_L35_mathematics_paper1.pdf> accessed 6 November 2016

6 Newton, P., 2003. The defensibility of national curriculum assessment in England. *Research Papers in Education*, 18(2), pp.101–127

7 Koretz, D., 2008. *Measuring up*. Cambridge, Massachusetts: Harvard University Press, p.163

8 *Ibid*. p.43

9 Pearson, 2010. *Edexcel GCSE Mathematics B Unit 1: Statistics and Probability (Calculator)*, 9 November, question 14 <https://qualifications.pearson.com/content/dam/pdf/GCSE/Mathematics%20B/2010/Exam%20materials/5MB1H_01_que_20101109.pdf> accessed 6 November 2016

10 Willingham, D.T., 2007. Critical thinking. *American Educator*, Summer 2007 <http://www.aft.org/sites/default/files/periodicals/Crit_Thinking.pdf> accessed 6 November 2016

11 Wiliam, D., 2000. *Integrating Summative and Formative Functions of Assessment*. Keynote address to the European Association for Educational Assessment, Prague, Czech Republic

12 Standards and Testing Agency, 2016. *Scaled scores at key stage 2* <https://www.gov.uk/guidance/scaled-scores-at-key-stage-2> accessed 6 November 2016

13 Melton, A.W., 1967. Repetition and retrieval from memory. *Science*, 158, p.532

14 Cepeda, N.J. et al., 2006. Distributed practice in verbal recall tasks: A review and quantitative synthesis, *Psychological Bulletin*, 132(3), p.354

15 Hodgson, A and Spours, K, 2003. *Beyond A Levels: Curriculum 2000 and the Reform of 14–19 Qualifications*. Abingdon: Psychology Press, pp.91–92

16 Wilde, S. et al., 2006. *Nuffield review higher education focus groups: Preliminary report*, p.8. See also the final report: Pring, R et al., 2009. *Education for All: The Future of Education and Training for 14-19 year olds*. Abingdon: Routledge

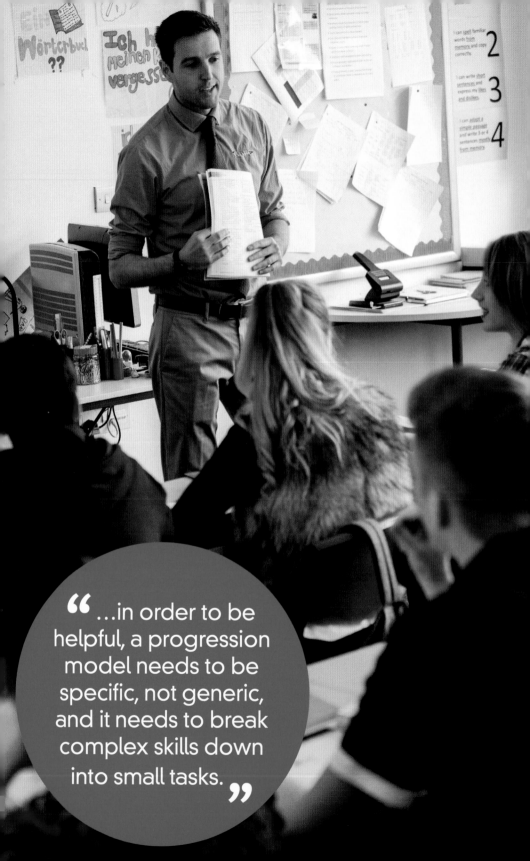

> " …in order to be helpful, a progression model needs to be specific, not generic, and it needs to break complex skills down into small tasks. "

Life after 'life after levels': creating a model of progression

6

In the previous two chapters we've looked at two in-school assessment systems which seem very different on the surface, but which are actually based on the same assumptions about how pupils improve. In the descriptor-based system, performance is measured by generic descriptions, not by specific tasks. In the exam-based system, performance is measured by specific tasks but progress is still measured by grades, even though the purpose of a grade is to describe performance, not to analyse it. As a result, even though the two systems look very different, they have many of the same flaws. They both:

- expect the same assessment to produce two very different inferences
- lead to overgrading and overtesting
- lead to unhelpful feedback
- lead to the measurement of formative progress with summative grades
- inadvertently encourage a focus on short-term performance and discourage long-term learning.

Even though national curriculum levels and the APP scheme have been abolished, and even though schools are free to develop their own assessment systems, we've seen that many of the new systems that have been developed are not fundamentally different. The opportunity of 'life after levels' has passed without any meaningful changes to the assessment systems that schools use. The rest of this book will suggest some more fundamental reforms to in-school assessment which could solve some of the problems of these systems. The next two chapters will look at ways in which formative and summative assessments could be improved, and the final chapter will put forward a system for integrating both types of assessment. The rest of this chapter will consider the importance of getting the right model of progression. No assessment system can succeed unless it is based on a clear and accurate understanding of how pupils make progress in different subjects.

Making progress

One of the major problems with the systems in the previous paragraph was that they expected different inferences to be made from the same assessment. So, one important principle is that assessments have to be selected and designed with reference to their purpose. Different assessments will serve different purposes; we cannot expect one assessment to produce all the inferences we need. Koretz makes this point in his analysis of portfolio-based assessment, which is similar to the descriptor-based assessment we looked at in Chapter 4:

> Policy-makers in the US often try to meet disparate goals with a
> single assessment. The various goals, however, may be in conflict.
> Portfolio assessment has attributes that make it particularly appealing
> to those who wish to use assessment and encourage richer instruction
> – for example, the authentic nature of some tasks, the reliance on
> large tasks, the lack of standardisation, and the close integration
> of assessment with instruction. But some of these attributes may

undermine the ability of the assessments to provide performance data
of comparable meaning across large numbers of schools. One size may
not fit all.

Koretz, D., *Large-scale Portfolio Assessments in the US*, p.332

We cannot rely on just one assessment or one style of assessment for all the assessment information we need. However, this is not to say we should completely separate assessments designed for formative and summative purposes. After all, improvements on formative assessments do lead, ultimately, to improvements on summative assessments. For example, pupils who get faster at decoding phonemes do become better readers; those who establish a clear sequence of historical events do get better at source analysis.

Although it is difficult to make formative and summative inferences from the same assessment, there still needs to be a link between them. This principle is well understood in sport; when a coach sets up a passing drill for a football team, or a physiotherapist designs a new stretching regime for a runner, they are deliberately choosing tasks that do not look like the final game or race for which the athlete is training. However, they are also deliberately choosing tasks that they think will improve a particular aspect of the team or the athlete's final performance. The drill and the final performance are different and separate, but they are linked. The link between them is what Wiliam calls a model of progression:

To be effective as a recipe for future action, the future action must be
designed so as to progress learning. In other words, the feedback must
embody a model of progression, and here, again, is where much coaching
in athletics programs is well designed. It is not enough to clarify the
current state and the goal state. The coach has to design a series of
activities that will move athletes from their current state to the goal state.

Wiliam, D., *Embedded formative assessment*, p.122

A good assessment system must not only clarify the current state and the goal state, which it can do through the use of summative assessments, but it must also establish a path between the two: the model of progression. An assessment system has to make clear the link between the activities being done in the individual lessons, the summative exams that come at the end, and the wider domain of expertise the exam is sampling from. The rest of this chapter will consider how best we can communicate, create and measure the model of progression.

Communicating the model of progression

Before we think about creating models of progression in different subjects, we need to think first about how they can be defined and communicated. We've seen in Chapters 4 and 5 that the dominant means of communicating models of progression are prose statements or exam specifications and past papers. These methods of communication are a part of the problem: they are not specific or detailed enough. An alternative medium which is more specific and detailed is the textbook.

Textbooks include some prose, of course, but they also include diagrams, illustrations, and, perhaps most importantly, examples and questions which are able to communicate meaning with precision. In Chapter 4, we looked at Kuhn's argument about the importance of examples in communicating scientific meaning: he said that students acquire scientific understanding by acquiring the 'arsenal of exemplars' that feature in textbooks.[1] More recently, a similar point about the importance of textbooks has been made by Tim Oates, Group Director at Cambridge Assessment. In a paper from 2010, he spoke about the importance of curriculum coherence, a similar concept to the model of progression we have been discussing:

The term 'coherence' does not carry the meaning typically associated with a 'broad and balanced curriculum' but is a highly precise technical term: a national curriculum should have content arranged in an order which is securely based in evidence associated with age-related progression, and all elements of the system (content, assessment, pedagogy, teacher training, teaching materials, incentives and drivers etc) should all line up and act in a concerted way to deliver public goods (Schmidt W & Prawat R 2006).

Oates, T., Could do better, p.4

In a later paper, Oates noted that many high-performing education systems used textbooks to create such coherence. Although textbooks have a slightly old-fashioned and outdated reputation in England, they offer an effective and detailed way of communicating a progression model and creating curriculum coherence. Oates's research found that the very best textbooks offered the following advantages:[2]

- underpinned by well-grounded learning theory and theory regarding subject-specific content
- clear delineation of content – a precise focus on key concepts and knowledge
- coherent learning progressions within the subject
- stimulation and support of learner reflection
- varied application of concepts and principles – 'expansive application'
- control of surface and structural features of texts to ensure consistency with underpinning learning theory.

Unfortunately, he also noted that few of these high-quality textbooks were being used in England:

The narrow instrumentalism displayed by many textbooks in England and the neglect of structured materials in favour of the use of

'worksheets' stands in stark contrast to these high-quality materials
and the manner in which they are used – by both teachers and pupils.

Oates, T., *Why textbooks count: A policy paper*, p.5

A 2011 survey of primary maths teachers found that only 10% of teachers in England said that they used textbooks as a basis for instruction. In Finland and Singapore, two of the world's best-performing education systems, the equivalent percentages were 95% and 70%.[3]

When thinking about what a model of progression should look like, we need to think less about sheets of paper and more about a set of textbooks. Of course, modern technology means that textbooks no longer have to be actual books. Digital textbooks can include the prose and examples of the traditional textbook and supplement these with video and audio material. They can also be interactive: instead of pupils responding to textbook questions on paper, they can answer them on a computer or tablet and receive instant feedback.

In the final chapter, I will give a brief sketch of what such a technology-enhanced model of progression might look like. However, such a system is a long way off, and the bulk of the rest of this book will look at technologically simpler methods of creating a progression model and establishing assessments within it. And, whether one chooses a paper or digital textbook, the important thing to note is that a textbook is more likely to result in the right model of progression than an exam specification or an APP-style grid.

Creating the right model of progression

If we accept that a textbook, together with supporting material such as a teacher guide, is a better way of communicating a model of progression, then how do we first go about creating or selecting a model? We've already seen two important principles: in order to be helpful, a progression model needs to be specific, not generic, and it needs to break complex skills down into small tasks that do not overload pupils' limited working memories. As the progression model builds, pupils will be able to manage more complex tasks because they have memorised and automated the initial steps, but the progression model must start with these initial basics. These are principles that are consistent across a number of subjects and are the result of our limited working memories. However, precisely because the progression model must be specific, it will look different in different subjects and, indeed, even for different concepts within the same subject. A progression model requires teachers to make decisions about what tasks are most likely to lead to the attainment of the end goal in that particular subject. In some subjects, there is a lot of research which can help with making these decisions, and even some detailed programmes which effectively are progression models in their own right.

Before we look at these, it is worth clarifying what the end goal or final aim of education should be. We said in the first chapter that, in general, the goals of education were less disputed than we might think. Most people would agree, for example, with the various versions of the national curriculum which say that, amongst other things, the aims of the English curriculum are to develop pupils' ability to communicate, and to instil in them a love of reading. We should begin with these curriculum aims when planning our progression model, and it is incredibly important that we continue to use these as our aims, rather than exam success. Exams are only samples from wider domains, and because of this, there will always be ways of doing well on them that do not lead to genuine learning. As long as we set our end goal as mastery of a particular domain, then exams will be valid measures of that goal.

The moment we start to target the exam, then the exam will stop being a valid measure. This is true not just in education, but in other areas. Goodhart's Law, named after the UK economist Charles Goodhart, states that when a measure becomes a target, it loses value as a measure. Goodhart came up with the idea when he saw the distortions that happened after the UK government targeted the supply of money in the economy.[4] In the US, Campbell's Law expresses a similar idea. If our end goal is success on an exam, we will end up with a progression model which leads to exam success, but not to the wider goals we really want. This is the fundamental problem with teaching to the test: tests are not direct measures of the domain, only samples. Teaching to the test is therefore a major threat to the validity of most of the inferences we want to make. The next few paragraphs will consider this issue in more depth, and draw heavily on research done by Koretz.[5–7]

Additional threats to validity — teaching to the test

Throughout the past few chapters, we have encountered lots of different threats to the validity of the inferences we want to make from exams: cramming, for example, which boosts short-term performance, not long-term learning. But there are other, subtler, threats to validity, which may not immediately seem as though they are that damaging. Indeed, in some cases, they may even seem to represent good practice. Take the common practice of coaching in the details of the exam question. Most UK exam textbooks devote large amounts of space to preparing pupils to answer various types of questions: 8-mark questions such as, 'The use of propaganda was the main reason the Nazis were able to control the German people. How far do you agree with this view?' or 16-mark questions such as, 'The Wall Street Crash was the main reason Hitler got into power. Do you agree?'[8] This is one of the features of such textbooks that led Oates to criticize them for having 'highly instrumental approaches to learning, oriented towards obtaining specific examination grades.'[2] These 8-mark and 16-mark questions are features of the sample, not the domain. They do not correspond to the types of problems pupils will face in real life so, if pupils have focused excessively on these types of questions, it will compromise the validity of those results. What counts as 'excessive focus'? To a certain extent, Koretz says, some coaching in how to answer these specific problems will actually increase the validity of exam scores:

> *If the format or content of a test is sufficiently unfamiliar, a modest amount of coaching may even increase the validity of scores. For example, the first time young students are given a test that requires filling in bubbles on an optical scanning sheet, it is worth spending a very short time familiarizing them with this procedure before they start the test.*
>
> Koretz, D., *Measuring Up*, p.255

Koretz also says that, most of the time, this kind of coaching 'either wastes time or inflates scores.' What is the difference between legitimate coaching that increases the validity of the exam score, and coaching that starts to compromise it?

> *Inflation occurs when coaching generates gains that are limited to a specific test – or to others that are very similar – and that do not generalize well to other tests of the same domain or to performance in real life.*
>
> Koretz, D., *Measuring Up*, p.255

To investigate this problem, Koretz carried out a study where he compared the results that the same group of pupils got on two different maths tests. Although the tests were different, they were both samples from the same domain, and indeed were both 'traditional, standardized, multiple-choice achievement tests...they differed only in details.'[9] One of the tests was the official high-stakes test by which schools were judged. Koretz found that pupils did half an academic year better on the official high-stakes test than on the other test, which was nevertheless sampling from the same domain. This, therefore, is an example of score inflation, because the pupils' performance on the official test was limited to that test, and was not reflected in their scores on other tests. Other research by

Koretz has found similar patterns elsewhere.[6–7] No similar research has been carried out in England, but one suggestive piece of data is found in Coe's analysis of exam performance which we looked at in Chapter 1.[10] He shows that the dramatic improvements in exam performance over the last thirty years have not been borne out by equivalent improvements on other tests, that is, on other assessments of the same domain. For example, significant improvements in the pass rates for GCSE English and maths tests are not matched by equivalent improvements in the Programme for International Student Assessment (PISA) maths and reading tests. One possible explanation of this pattern of results is the practice of teaching to the test.

Koretz shows that one of the reasons why this kind of teaching to the test has come about in the US is because of an increase in high-stakes testing regimes.[9] Again, the UK has similar high-stakes testing systems, with schools, head teachers and teachers being held accountable for the results of their pupils on Key Stage 2 national tests (SATs), GCSEs and A levels. Not only that, but as we've seen, Ofsted also look at schools' own internal assessment data, effectively turning these into high-stakes tests as well. Koretz also argues that teaching to the test techniques tend to become popular when schools are expected to make very dramatic improvements over short periods of time, because it is hard to achieve such improvements in more legitimate ways.[9] Again, we have also seen this in our analysis: if pupils are graded every term, or even every few weeks, and dramatic improvements are expected over these short periods, then cramming and teaching to the test are probably the only methods that will provide such short-term improvements.

Whilst high-stakes testing regimes are undoubtedly one reason behind the increase in teaching to the test, another reason is the widespread misunderstanding of the difference between the sample and the domain. Koretz recounts many conversations with education officials who defended the kinds of practices outlined earlier. One US principal argued that her school's excellent test scores had been achieved by teaching to the test, but that this was fine because the test was measuring valuable skills and knowledge. Koretz goes so far as to call this argument 'nonsense'. In the UK, there is a similar misunderstanding of this vital point. One common response to England's improved GCSE scores but stagnant PISA scores is to claim that it is because pupils hadn't been taught to the PISA tests. Sir John Rowling, the chair of the PiXL club, has suggested that the difference between the GCSE and PISA scores can be explained by this fact: if we want to improve on the PISA tests, then we should direct instruction to them.[11] But the PISA tests of mathematics, literacy and science are drawing from the same domains as the GCSEs in those subjects. If pupils are performing far better on the latter than the former, it calls into question the validity of the most common inferences we make about GCSEs.

The difference between teaching to the test and the domain was illustrated for me by a comment made by one of my A-level English literature students. The first question in this exam required students to write a close analysis of one of a dozen Thomas Hardy poems listed in the specification. I had written the students a couple of model essays on some of the poems. A student asked me if I could write model essays for all of the poems in the specification. They could then memorise these model essays and reproduce them in the exam. From the point of view of efficiency, she was probably right. If one defines the end goal as success in an exam, then perhaps the most efficient way of ensuring success for all pupils in such an exam would be to do something similar. Of course, this is an extreme example, but it illustrates the difference between preparing pupils to understand the wider domain, and preparing them to pass a test. However well-designed a test is, there will always be alternative methods of passing it that do not involve mastering the domain it is based on and, if a test is poorly designed, such alternative methods may even be more efficient.

This example also illustrates the difference between memorising the right thing and memorising the wrong thing. Whilst I thought it was a bad idea for pupils to memorise model essays, I did expect pupils to memorise quotations from Hardy's poems, even though it was an open-book exam. I expected this because I felt it could help them with two of the important aims of the English curriculum: using evidence to support opinion, and appreciating poetry. Memorising quotations would help to reduce the load on working memory as they justified their opinion about Hardy's poetry. It would also help them to spot patterns and links when reading poetry in the future, long after the exam was over. Memorising lines of poetry, therefore, helps pupils to move towards the end goals of the English curriculum in ways which are not achieved by memorising model essays.

Choosing what to remember

How should we make decisions about what knowledge is worth remembering, and what isn't? Willingham proposes three categories of content that are particularly worth practising and remembering:[12]

- The core skills and knowledge that will be used again and again.
- The knowledge that students need to know well in the short term to enable long-term retention of key concepts. In this case, short-term overlearning is merited.
- The knowledge we believe is important enough that students should remember it later in life.

For Willingham, 'simple maths facts' belong to the first category. Number bonds and times tables recur in all kinds of other maths problems, so it is worth learning them. However, we can also see from this that there is less value to be gained from memorising some other maths facts. Primary maths teachers do not get their students to memorise maths facts of the type 32 × 76, or 54 × 62. This is because these facts do not appear in lots of other problems and do not form the basis of later maths skill. This is similar to the difference between memorising lines of Hardy's poetry and memorising model essays.

Remembering some things will create meaning. Remembering others will not create meaning. Whether memorisation does create meaning is dependent on the content of what is memorised. It is also dependent on the entire curriculum and the series of lessons. The same lesson may or may not create meaning, depending on the sequence it is a part of. For example, we've seen that memorising times tables helps pupils to do maths, so a lesson that focuses on the 6 times table is perfectly justified as a path to creating meaning. However, suppose that, for whatever reason, a teacher only ever taught a single lesson on the 6 times tables. This, in isolation, would not be effective at creating meaning. The same lesson is more or less effective depending on the sequence of lessons it is a part of. It is perhaps for this reason that individual lesson observations can be so misleading. It is possible for one lesson to be highly effective if it is part of one sequence, and highly ineffective if it is part of another. It is also for this reason that lessons which do involve the decontextualisation and memorisation of small facts can appear so atomised and meaningless: they appear this way because they are being viewed out of the context of the progression model.

Therefore, in establishing a progression model we first have to establish what it is we want a pupil to be able to achieve. We have to define this in terms of the fundamental concepts we want them to master, not in terms of exam success. Once we have done that, then we can look at the research which explains how best to achieve such an aim and exactly what small and specific chunks pupils need to learn. To a certain extent, particularly in some subjects, there are genuinely competing visions of what it is we want pupils to achieve. In many subjects, however, there is broad agreement over what we want pupils to achieve and the debate is about the most effective progression model which will achieve those aims. Whereas the debate about aims is essentially one of values and cannot therefore be resolved by research, the debate about methods can be: even if, in some subjects such as history, geography and religious studies, extensive research doesn't yet exist.

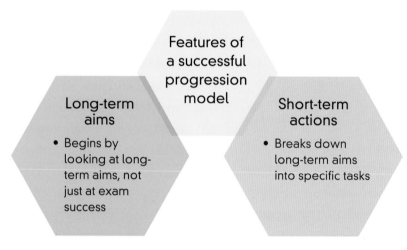

Figure 6.1: Features of a successful progression model

Examples of progression models

One area where a lot of research does exist is reading; we know that teaching pupils the correspondence between certain patterns of letters and the sounds they represent is vital.[13] These letter-sound correspondences are perhaps analogous to times tables in maths, in that they are fundamental building blocks which enable so much else. In many reading programmes, pupils learn to recognise these correspondences so they are automatic and fluent; pupils are then able to use them to decode any new word they come across.[14] As well as decoding, another vital part of the reading progression model is vocabulary, but learning vocabulary is different from learning to decode in a couple of ways. There are only 26 letters in the English language, and only 44 phonemes, or units of sound, but there are tens of thousands of words. Also, the meanings of words are learnt in a different way from phonemes: in certain circumstances, we can implicitly learn the meaning of new words in a way that we cannot learn the phonetic code.[15]

As a result, the reading researcher Isobel Beck recommends teaching about 400 words a year for the first ten years of education. Specifically, she recommends teaching a set of words which she calls 'Tier Two' words.[16] Tier One words are basic, everyday words that you can rely on all pupils knowing already: for example, 'table', 'chair' and 'happy'. Tier Three words are rare or subject-specific words, that pupils will not encounter frequently in spoken or written language: words like 'filibuster', 'aorta', or 'bruit'. In contrast with these, Tier Two words are common in prose but are less common in everyday speech: words such as 'eradicate', 'inevitable', 'restrict', 'variation' and 'industrious'. We cannot rely on pupils picking them up from everyday interactions, but if pupils are to become fluent readers of sophisticated texts, they are vital. They are also the kinds of words that will enable pupils to learn new words. The research on vocabulary also recommends that pupils learn examples of vocabulary rather than definitions: as we've seen again and again, prose definitions are paradoxically only helpful when you know what they mean already.[17]

This body of research enables teachers to make a decision about what knowledge is most worthwhile, what is less valuable, and what the best method of teaching it is. Lots of programmes for teaching phonics exist already, most of which represent a research-based progression model.[14] Nothing similar exists for teaching vocabulary, but one could imagine a similar series of textbooks or set of resources which aimed to teach 400 Tier Two words a year from years 1–9; that's the equivalent of about 10 words per school week.

Up to this point, many of our examples have focused on the very basic building blocks of the progression model. That's because these basic building blocks are often the hardest to infer if we only look at final performance, and because they are the ones that expert adults are so likely to take for granted. As pupils progress through a subject and master the smaller building blocks, they are able to deal with larger tasks. But even at these more advanced levels, the same kind of decomposed and decontextualised approach can work.

For example, once pupils have learned to read and write to a good standard, one way of teaching style and creativity would be to teach a series of lessons on rhetorical figures. In his book *The Elements of Eloquence*, Mark Forsyth lists and exemplifies a series of such figures, and defends the isolated teaching of them. He notes that the figures of rhetoric 'are formulas, formulas that you can learn from a book' and shows that when such figures were developed by the ancient Greeks, 'all that [they] were doing was noting down the best and most memorable phrases they heard, and working out what the structures were, in much the same way that when you or I eat a particularly delicious meal, we might ask for the recipe.'[18] It would be possible to imagine a textbook based on the rhetorical figures included in Forsyth's book, with each figure being expanded into a lesson that required pupils to identify examples of each one and then use it in a sentence or paragraph of their own. In fact, something like this used to exist: one of the most popular textbooks in England in the 16th century was Johannes Susenbrotus' guide to rhetorical techniques, *Epitome Troporum Ac Schematum*. It was almost certainly used at the school Shakespeare attended, as many of its stock phrases and examples are used in his plays.[19]

One other point to remember is that, whilst this discussion has been framed in terms of subjects, subjects may not always be the best way of thinking about progression models. Though subjects are a useful way of organising knowledge, they are not the only way. Some traditional school subjects consist of quite arbitrary content: the school subject of English, for example, includes instruction in the use of language as well as in the appreciation of literature. The school subject of geography combines human geography, which is perhaps closer to history in its approach, with physical geography, which is closer to the sciences. In many countries the content that is included in England's geography curriculum appears instead in history and biology curricula.

Perhaps the best way of creating a progression model, therefore, is to think in terms of the important concepts that we want pupils to acquire and the things we want them to be able to achieve at the end of their time in education. Doing this will also help us to see where some important aims cut across subject boundaries. For example, many important concepts in chemistry and physics depend on the knowledge taught in maths lessons. The knowledge and vocabulary taught in almost every lesson will help to improve reading ability. In particular, studies have shown that basic historical and geographical information has a significant impact on a pupil's ability to comprehend broadsheet newspaper articles.[20–21] If we think that being able to comprehend such articles is an important aim of education (and we may not) then we may also decide that some of the knowledge needed to develop such a skill is best taught in the history and geography curricula, not just in the English curriculum, and that the aims of history and geography curricula are therefore extended to include this.

Measuring the model of progression

Assuming we do build the right progression model, what is the most useful and accurate way of measuring progress within it? Assessment systems that are based on the idea of generic skill, like the two we looked at in Chapters 4 and 5, will always end up grading pupils very frequently. This is because, if you conceive of skill as something generic, then the differences between the types of activities you do in class and the types you do in the exam are just ones of degree, not of kind. As a result, they will be measured using the same scale and it will make sense to measure them very frequently to see if progress is being made.

The best analogy for this kind of measurement is measuring height. You can use the same tape measure and the same scale to measure a 4-year-old as you can to measure a 16-year-old. The method stays the same even as the child grows. You can also use the same scale to measure progress over time and, if you have a tape measure with small enough divisions, you can measure progress over quite short periods of time. This was ultimately why people started using grades in every lesson, and why the desire for subgrades and sublevels came about: people saw them as the millimetres and centimetres that made up the metres of progress. And, if you subscribe to this model, then ever finer subdivisions of grades are a perfectly good idea: they will allow you to measure the precise amounts of progress that are added in each lesson. It would be possible to say that after a week of lessons a pupil had added x% of a GCSE grade, or z fraction of a sublevel.

As we have seen, learning is not actually like this. Complex skills are made up of many different elements and those distinct elements all look very different and cannot be measured with the same scale. Learning is multidimensional, not unidimensional; comparing educational measurement to the measurement of height is convenient, but it is profoundly misleading. Instead of thinking about one scale that can be subdivided, we need to think about several scales that are related to each other.

A better metaphor for educational progress, therefore, is training for a marathon. Marathon runners measure their overall time in hours and minutes. In order to get better at running marathons, most coaches and marathon runners have progression models consisting of activities that will help them run faster.[22] Some of these activities are quite similar to the marathon itself or are just shorter versions of the marathon. For example, the coach might recommend that the runner should manage a long run of at least 21 miles a few weeks before the race itself, or they might recommend a half-marathon, which is also measured in hours and minutes. This might be the equivalent of a teacher recommending that a student does a full or partial mock exam in the months leading up to a terminal exam.

It is important to note that a running coach will also recommend other activities which do not involve running very long distances, as well as some which do not involve running at all, such as strength and conditioning exercises. It would obviously not make sense to measure these activities in the same way as the marathon. Instead, the coach might record the amount of weight the runner is able to lift, the number of repetitions of exercises they are able to complete, or even whether they are – or are not – able to complete certain exercises at all. All of these activities are the equivalent of classroom activities that help to develop skill: the vocabulary instruction, the multiple-choice quiz, the plenary activity, and so on. They are also similar to these classroom activities in that they don't just allow you to measure progress: they actually help pupils to make progress. In the same way that the act of trying to remember a word helps consolidate that memory, the act of holding the plank position, for example, helps to build core strength.

When all these very different measures are compared, it is possible to tease out some patterns between them. There are very good data sets which compare marathon times with times over shorter distances. For example, a runner who is aiming to complete a 4-hour marathon might expect to do a half-marathon in about 1 hour and 54 minutes and, when training, to do ten 800-metre repetitions in four minutes each.[23] There is also quite a bit of research on the types of strength and conditioning exercises long-distance runners need to do: generally, runners need to build up their core strength so they can maintain their running form over long distances. One paper recommends, among other exercises, that runners should try to hold a side plank position 'for 20sec, working up to one minute holds for two to three repetitions.'[24] Of course, if a runner does work up to this standard, it is not guaranteed that they will definitely run a faster marathon. An improvement of 10 seconds on the side plank does not equate to a set improvement of time on the marathon. Just as we shouldn't measure progress in individual lessons with fractions of grades, so it doesn't make sense to measure the time an athlete can hold a plank for as a fraction of a marathon time. The links between each training activity and the final performance are probabilistic, not deterministic: they make it more likely a runner will run faster, but they do not guarantee it.

Similarly, whilst each individual training element is important, on its own it can look quite insignificant or trivial: clearly, if someone training for a marathon only ever did strength and conditioning exercises or 800-metre repetitions, they would not be able to run a marathon very quickly. Still, the strength and conditioning can have an impact disproportionate to the time spent on it: successful marathon runners may well spend the bulk of their training time running, but the smaller amounts of time they spend on strength and conditioning are vital in preventing injury and enabling such heavy running loads.[25] Just as we've seen that overusing summative exam tasks and grades can impede learning, focussing too much on the marathon and the final marathon time would also be risky. Training for a marathon by running marathons would lead to lots of injuries, particularly for beginners.

Modern marathon training programmes do not consist of just one activity, but are made up of many different complementary elements. Improvements in training programmes have led to the world-record marathon time improving dramatically over the course of a century, and have also allowed hundreds of thousands of amateur runners to participate in marathon running and improve their times. As Ericsson shows, 'the fastest time for the marathon in the 1896 Olympic Games was just a minute faster than the required entry time in large marathon races such as the Boston Marathon'.[26] He attributes such improvements in these and other athletic disciplines mainly to 'the increase in amount of preparation and training and improvements in training methods'.[27]

What this suggests is that we need different scales and different types of assessment for the different elements we want to assess, and we need to recognise that the links between the different scales and tasks will be probabilistic, not deterministic. In the next two chapters, we will look at this issue in closer detail, and suggest some principles that can help us to choose the right assessments.

Notes

1 Kuhn, T.S., 2011. Second Thoughts on Paradigms. In *The Essential Tension: Selected Studies in Scientific Tradition and Change*. Chicago: University of Chicago Press, pp.293–320

2 Oates, T., 2014. *Why textbooks count: A policy paper*. Cambridge: University of Cambridge Local Examinations Syndicate, pp.4–6

3 Mullis, I.V.S., Martin, M.O., Foy, P. and Alka, A, 2012. *TIMSS 2011 International Results in Mathematics*. Chestnut Hill, Massachusetts: TIMSS & PIRLS International Study Center, Lynch School of Education, Boston College, p.392

4 Chrystal, K.A and Mizen, P.D., 2003. Goodhart's Law: its origins, meaning and implications for monetary policy. In Mizen, P., ed., *Central Banking, Monetary Theory and Practice: Essays in Honour of Charles Goodhart Vol. 1*. Cheltenham: Edward Elgar Publishing, pp.221–243

5 Koretz, D., 2008. *Measuring Up*, Cambridge: Harvard University Press, Chapter 10

6 Koretz, D.M., Linn, R.L, Dunbar, S.B. and Shepard, L.A, 1991. *The Effects of High-Stakes Testing On Achievement: Preliminary Findings About Generalization Across Tests*. Paper presented at the annual meeting of the American Educational Research Association, Chicago

7 Koretz, D.M. and Barron, S.I., 1998. *The validity of gains in scores on the Kentucky Instructional Results Information System (KIRIS)*. Santa Monica, California: Rand

8 For example, three major exam boards offer a history GCSE unit on Germany from 1919–1945, but no generic textbook covers this period. Instead, the Schools History Project have produced three different textbooks, one for each exam board. The example 16-mark question is taken from Culpin, C. and Banham, D., 2011. *Edexcel Germany 1919–1945 for SHP GCSE*. London: Hodder Education, p.45. The 8-mark question is taken from Culpin, C. and Banham, D., 2011. *OCR Germany 1919–1945 for SHP GCSE*. London: Hodder Education, p.60

9 Koretz, D., 2008. *Measuring Up*. Cambridge: Harvard University Press, pp.243–44, 250, 254

10 Coe, R, 2013. *Improving Education: A triumph of hope over experience*. Durham: Centre for Evaluation and Monitoring, Durham University, p.10

11 Stewart, W., 2013. England must better prepare pupils for Pisa tests to improve its ranking, heads' leader says. *Times Educational Supplement*, 2 December <https://news.tes.co.uk/b/news/2013/11/29/england-must-prepare-pupils-for-pisa-tests-to-improve-its-rankings.aspx> accessed 3 March 2015

12 Willingham, D.T., 2004. Practice Makes Perfect—But Only If You Practice Beyond the Point of Perfection. *American Educator*, Spring 2004 <http://www.aft.org/periodical/american-educator/spring-2004/ask-cognitive-scientist> accessed 6 November 2016

13 McGuinness, D., 2006. *Early Reading Instruction: What Science Really Tells Us about How to Teach Reading*. Cambridge, Massachusetts: MIT Press

14   See, for example: Read Write Inc <https://global.oup.com/education/content/primary/series/rwi/?region=uk>; Jolly Phonics <http://jollylearning.co.uk/overview-about-jolly-phonics/>; Sounds-Write <http://www.sounds-write.co.uk>; Sound Foundations <http://www.soundfoundations.co.uk> all accessed 6 November 2016

15   Hirsch Jr., E.D., 2006. *The Knowledge Deficit: Closing the Shocking Education Gap for American Children.* Boston: Houghton Mifflin, pp.61–65

16   Beck, I.L., McKeown M.G. and Kucan, L, 2013. *Bringing words to life: Robust Vocabulary Instruction* (second edition). New York: The Guilford Press, pp.8–10

17   Miller, G.A and Gildea, P.M., 1987. How Children Learn Words. *Scientific American,* 257, pp.94–99

18   Forsyth, M., 2013. *The elements of eloquence: How to turn the perfect English phrase.* London: Icon Books Ltd, p.4

19   Baldwin, T.W., 1944. *William Shakspere's Small Latine & Lesse Greeke. Vol. 2.* Chicago: University of Illinois Press, pp.138–148

20   Willinsky, J., 1998. *The Vocabulary of Cultural Literacy in a Newspaper of Substance.* Paper presented at the Annual Meeting of the National Reading Conference, 29 November–3 December 1988, Tucson, Arizona

21   Hirsch E.D., Kett, J.F. and Trefil, J.S., 2002. *The New Dictionary of Cultural Literacy.* Boston: Houghton Mifflin

22   See, for example: Hilditch, G., 2014. *Marathon and Half Marathon: A Training Guide* (second edition). Malborough: Crowood Press

23   These predictions were made with the McMillan Running Calculator <https://www.mcmillanrunning.com> accessed 6 November 2016

24   Fredericson, M. and Moore, T., 2005. Muscular balance, core stability, and injury prevention for middle-and long-distance runners. *Physical Medicine and Rehabilitation Clinics of North America,* 16(3), pp.669–689

25   Pavey, J., 2009. Strength training. *The Guardian,* 10 January <https://www.theguardian.com/lifeandstyle/2009/jan/10/strength-training-running> accessed 6 November 2016

26   Ericsson, KA, Krampe, RT. and Tesch-Römer, C, 1993. The Role of Deliberate Practice in the Acquisition of Expert Performance. *Psychological Review,* 100, pp.363–406

27   Ericsson, KA, 1990. Peak performance and age: An examination of peak performance in sports. In Baltes, P. and M., eds. *Successful Aging: Perspectives from the Behavioral Sciences,* pp.164–196

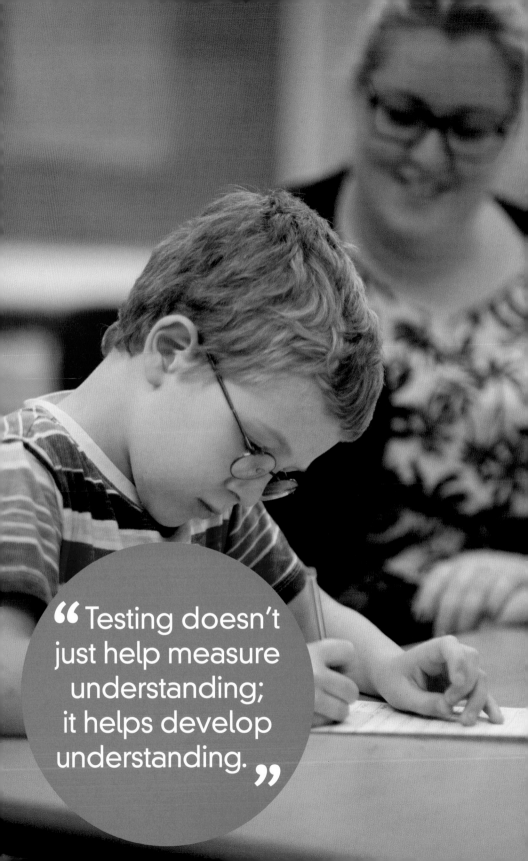

"Testing doesn't just help measure understanding; it helps develop understanding."

Improving formative assessments

Once a progression model is established, what should the formative assessments within it look like, and how should they be recorded? We've seen in previous chapters that the aim of formative assessments should be to identify useful next steps for the teacher and pupil. Based on this, here are some suggestions about the features of formative assessments. They should be:

- specific
- frequent
- repetitive
- recorded as raw marks.

In the rest of this chapter, we will consider each of these in turn.

Specificity

We've seen throughout the previous chapters how important it is for teaching, assessments and feedback to be specific. Specific questions allow teachers to diagnose exactly what a pupil's strengths and weaknesses are, and they make it easy, even obvious, to work out what to do next, whereas open and complex questions like essays or real-world problems are not particularly well-suited to this. Short-answer and multiple-choice questions, by contrast, can be very precise.

Multiple-choice questions are particularly useful, but they have an undeserved bad reputation, so the next few paragraphs will focus on their strengths. A couple of examples will show how multiple-choice questions are able to be very precise; how they are easy to analyse; how they are capable, contrary to many people's beliefs, of assessing difficult material in a range of subjects; and how they make it easy to give meaningful feedback.

The usefulness of multiple-choice questions

First, multiple-choice questions are able to be very precise and to focus on one small aspect of a topic. Take the following question:

> **How did the Soviet totalitarian system under Stalin differ from that of Hitler and Mussolini?**

This question could easily be set as an essay question. If that were the case, then, as we have seen, it might give us a good idea of how well our pupils were doing but not necessarily what they needed to work on next. In actual fact, this question was set as a multiple-choice item as part of a Canadian school-leaving exam. The four answer options were as follows:[1]

> **How did the Soviet totalitarian system under Stalin differ from that of Hitler and Mussolini?**
>
> **a)** It built up armed forces.
> **b)** It took away human rights.
> **c)** It made trade unions illegal.
> **d)** It abolished private land ownership.

The question requires the same kind of thinking as the essay question, but in a more targeted way which makes the answer easier to interpret. For example, if a pupil answers with options 'a' or 'b', they have not understood two of the most fundamental aspects of Hitler and Mussolini's dictatorships. Option 'c' is perhaps the more interesting distractor and the one that many pupils may choose. It is easy to see why pupils might make this error: in theory, if not in practice, communism was supportive of trade unions, so pupils with a relatively superficial idea of these dictators might think this is the answer. The correct answer, 'd', is also well chosen because the concept of abolishing private land ownership is an unfamiliar and abstract one which many pupils in the modern West struggle to understand.

If this question had been set as an essay and not as a multiple-choice question, it would have been much harder to make such inferences. A pupil with a shaky understanding of the role of trade unions in the Soviet Union might have written an essay that didn't mention trade unions or private property at all, perhaps focussing instead on Hitler's aggression or the Holocaust. It would therefore have been impossible for the teacher to have inferred much about their understanding of two vital concepts. Of course, there are other important aspects of the interwar dictatorships that this question does not address, but one other advantage of multiple-choice questions is that compared to essays, they are quick to answer and to mark. Twenty multiple-choice questions of this type on this topic would give a teacher a far better understanding of a pupil's specific strengths and weaknesses than one essay, and it would probably still take less time for teachers to mark and give feedback, as well as less time for pupils to complete.

A criticism of such questions is that they make it easy for pupils to guess the answer, but this risk can be mitigated in several different ways. You can increase the number of distractors, making it less likely that a guess will be right. You can increase the number of questions: a pupil might get lucky once or twice, but they are unlikely to get lucky five or ten times. You can also include more than one right answer, as in this example:

> **Which of the following are living things?**
> **a)** An oak tree
> **b)** A volcano
> **c)** A car
> **d)** A computer
> **e)** A chicken

With this question, the pupil does not know how many of the distractors are correct, which means their chances of guessing correctly are just 1 in 32. If a pupil is asked to answer just two questions like this, then the likelihood of them guessing and getting each question right is already less than 1 in 1000.

One other way of mitigating this problem for one-off questions in the classroom is to analyse the result of a question at the level of the class, not at the level of the individual. If one pupil gives the right answer to a true or false question, there is the possibility that they have guessed, with a 1 in 2 chance of success. But if you give the same question to just 10 pupils, and they all guess the answer, the likelihood of them all being correct is less than 1 in 1000.

One advantage of the precision and specificity of multiple-choice questions is that they are able to target misconceptions very effectively. In maths and science, for example, there are a number of misconceptions with which many pupils struggle, and lots of academic work has been carried out to identify them and work out the best way to overcome them.[2–5] Misconceptions are an important part of a progression model because often they involve particularly tricky and fundamental concepts, without which pupils cannot progress.

For example, in maths, there are a lot of misconceptions about percentages. Some pupils confuse calculating percentages with division. They are often encouraged in this misconception by the fact that when you are calculating 10% of something, you can divide by 10. The following question and distractors are designed to see if pupils have really understood how percentages work:

What is 20% of 300?
a) 30
b) 60
c) 15
d) 6000

If a pupil answers with 'c', the teacher can make a fairly good inference that she is confusing percentages and division, or she is assuming that because you can calculate 10% of something by dividing by 10, you can calculate 20% by dividing by 20. Pupils who answer with 'a' might be very good at calculating 10%, but uncertain about how to calculate other percentages. And pupils who answer with 'd' might have confused percentages and multiplication.

This brings us to a second advantage of multiple-choice questions: they are very easy to analyse. If you have ten questions of the type shown, it is possible to record not just whether a pupil got each question right or wrong, but what distractor they chose. It's then possible to record all of the answers in a question-level analysis spreadsheet of the type we saw in Chapter 5. We saw that such analysis was less helpful when it is based on the range of questions typically found in a summative exam. However, when the analysis is done on a set of questions on one topic that has been recently taught, then it becomes much more helpful. If a teacher set 10 questions like the ones shown, and a pupil got all 10 correct, then it is fair to assume that at that moment in time, at least, the pupil has understood how to calculate a percentage. Similarly, if on the question shown a pupil puts the equivalent of option 'c' for all 10 questions, then it is very likely that they have confused percentages and division. So in this case, the question-level analysis does allow for useful feedback to the teacher and pupil. This is particularly the case when the distractor the pupil chose is recorded, not just whether they got it right or wrong.

Another criticism of multiple-choice questions is that, while they are effective for simple tasks in subjects like maths and science, they are less effective with more sophisticated material and in subjects like English and history. The earlier question about the Soviet Union should show this is not the case, but another question taken from an undergraduate politics resource also demonstrates this:[6]

> **Liberal ideology…**
> **a)** was invented in the eighteenth century to serve the interests of the British Liberal Party.
> **b)** developed as a hostile response to the emergence of industrial capitalism.
> **c)** is a compromise between socialism and conservatism.
> **d)** is a long-established creed which focuses on individual freedom.

The questions in this resource are accompanied by some explanatory paragraphs showing why each option is right or wrong:

The correct answer is d. Liberalism predates the British Liberal Party, which was not known by that name until the mid-1800s (answer a). Far from being hostile to industrial capitalism (answer b), liberalism

is seen by some critics as an attempt to justify this economic system.
The ideology is certainly not a compromise between socialism and
conservatism; its focus on individual liberty makes it clearly distinct
from those ideologies.

Garner, R., Ferdinand, P. and Lawson, S., *Introduction to Politics*

This explanatory paragraph shows the final advantage of multiple-choice questions: they make it easy to give meaningful feedback. Instead of a teacher having to puzzle over an essay, make a shaky inference about the pupil's misconception and then think of a question that will target that misconception, they can prepare such feedback in advance based on the distractors. Once the feedback has been delivered, the teacher can then follow up with another set of similar questions to see if the pupil has understood this time round. Multiple-choice questions, together with this kind of in-depth, specific and precise feedback, can form a vital part of a progression model in any subject.

Frequency

So far, when we have looked at the positive effects of formative assessments on learning, we have tended to look at the way the information from the formative assessments is used. That is, we've looked at the indirect benefits of assessment: giving pupils a quiz on something they've just learned allows the teacher and pupil to see if the pupil has understood it or not, and then to act quickly in response to that information. As we've seen, this is very powerful. However, there is another, more direct, benefit to be gained from these kinds of quick assessments. Research shows that the act of recalling information from memory actually helps to strengthen the memory itself. That is, testing doesn't just help measure understanding; it helps develop understanding:

Testing not only measures knowledge, but also changes it, often greatly
improving retention of the tested knowledge. Taking a test on material

can have a greater positive effect on future retention of that material
than spending an equivalent amount of time restudying the material.

Roediger, H.L. and Karpicke, J.D., *The power of testing memory*, p.181

This effect is known as the testing effect, or the retrieval effect. Together with the indirect benefits to be gained from assessments, the testing effect is a powerful argument for increasing the amount of quizzing and assessment in the classroom. Many of the same researchers who have carried out studies into the testing effect have also carried out studies into the value of multiple-choice questions and have concluded that these are particularly effective ways to realise the benefits of the testing effect.[7–8]

Why is it that such formative assessments should be frequent, but summative assessments should be infrequent? If there is benefit to be had from frequent testing, surely it can apply to summative assessment too? Indeed, Roediger and Karpicke, two of the most prominent researchers in this field, are at pains to point out that the testing effect can apply to complex tasks.[9] However, when judging whether the testing effect will apply or not, the important difference is perhaps not about the complexity of the material, but about whether a task involves retrieval or not. It is the act of retrieving knowledge from long-term memory which strengthens the memory. If content is not in long-term memory to begin with, then pupils cannot retrieve it. Many of the tasks on summative exams will involve material that is not in long-term memory, particularly given the way that summative exams have to be designed to cater to a range of abilities. In these cases, pupils are not retrieving something from long-term memory but using problem-solving search, and, as we've seen, 'learners can engage in problem-solving activities for extended periods and learn almost nothing'.[10] In these cases, there is a risk of cognitive overload, as pupils are confronted with a great deal of new information which has to be processed in limited working memory.[11] This is a particular issue when pupils are confronted with texts that contain difficult vocabulary, or which assume prior knowledge: there only need to be a few unknown words in a text for a pupil's understanding to break down.[12]

Introducing desirable difficulties

Indeed, prior knowledge is an important consideration here. The power of the testing effect is that it introduces what Bjork terms a 'desirable difficulty' into learning.[13] Some difficulties are desirable and tests which require retrieval from memory are an example of this. One popular revision technique is to reread the material that will be on the test, but this is actually much less effective than self-testing. One plausible reason for this is that rereading is too easy: pupils can reread a text, feel familiar with the content, but not have really thought about it.[13] However, whilst some difficulties are desirable, some are undesirable, and an important factor in telling the difference is prior knowledge. In Bjork's words:

> *Before proceeding further, we need to emphasize the importance of the word desirable. Many difficulties are undesirable during instruction and forever after. Desirable difficulties, versus the array of undesirable difficulties, are desirable because they trigger encoding and retrieval processes that support learning, comprehension, and remembering. If, however, the learner does not have the background knowledge or skills to respond to them successfully, they become undesirable difficulties.*
>
> Bjork, E.L. and Bjork, R.A., *Making things hard on yourself, but in a good way*, p.58

Whether difficulties are desirable or not may therefore depend less on the difficulty of the material, and more on the prior knowledge of the individual. Again, we see the importance of viewing tasks and activities as part of a progression model instead of in isolation. The same task could help or hinder learning, depending on where it is placed in a curriculum. For example, introducing a new vocabulary word in the same lesson as introducing a new novel, a new set of characters, and a new literary technique might involve too many difficulties. Introducing the very same new word towards the middle of a unit of work, once pupils have a better understanding of the characters in the novel, could be much more effective.

When deciding what is or isn't a desirable difficulty, we also need to be aware of a number of cognitive biases that are likely to make teachers and pupils underestimate the difficulty of certain tasks. Adults, for example, can often underestimate their own knowledge and overestimate the knowledge of children. Once we have reached proficiency in an area, we often forget the effort and the specifics of the process which got us there.[14] Pupils and novices are subject to other sets of biases: for example, pupils often confuse familiarity with understanding.[15] Indeed, one of the reasons why the testing effect is such an effective method of study is that, unlike rereading or restudy of content, it makes it very clear if pupils have really understood something, or if they are just familiar with it.

We need to consider all of these factors when working out how pupils can benefit from the testing effect and desirable difficulties, and to be aware that tasks at the right level of difficulty may seem quite simple and superficial. We also need to remember how easily we forget things: it's because of this that we frequently need to repeat and restudy material we have already learned.

Repetition

We saw in Chapter 3 that one of the major threats to the validity of any formative inference is that performance is not learning. This is a huge problem, because many formative inferences need to be made quickly, using evidence from short-term performance, so that teachers can respond quickly. However, a pupil can perform well in the short term without having fully learnt something. This means that if we want to make an inference about whether a pupil needs more teaching on a particular topic, or whether they are ready to move on, then an assessment which takes place in or soon after the lesson cannot allow us to make a valid inference about that.

This problem can only be solved if we factor in information about the difference between performance and learning when we are making the formative inference: as Willingham says, 'anticipating the effect of forgetting dictates that we continue our practice beyond the mastery we desire.'[16] We have to remember that if a pupil gets a particular question right, that on its own does not provide us with a valid inference about whether they have truly learnt the concept being tested. In order to be able to make an inference about that, we have to use other information from previous assessments: to consider how many times pupils have studied and been tested on that topic in the past, and their performance on those questions too.

The progression model must also make this easier by building in the opportunity for repetition and consolidation, even if pupils get questions right the first time. As we've seen, perhaps the best way of building in this repetition and consolidation is through short classroom quizzes because, in these cases, the very act of trying to recall information will help to consolidate the memory. Research on the best way of sequencing such practice shows that it needs to be spaced out, or distributed, over time, rather than being 'massed' into a short period.[17–18] This would suggest that in the set of questions that pupils do at the end of the lesson or for homework, only some should be taken from that lesson's topic; others should recap topics from previous lessons. Spreading out questions like this is an example of spaced-practice, or distributed-practice. It's an alternative to massed-practice, or cramming.

With this distributed practise format, each lesson is followed by the usual number of practise problems, but only a few of these problems relate to the immediately preceding lesson. Additional problems of the same type might also appear once or twice in each of the next dozen assignments and once again after every fifth or tenth assignment thereafter.

Rohrer, D. and Taylor, K., *The effects of overlearning and distributed practise on the retention of mathematics knowledge*, p.1218

Therefore, repetition of material and spaced practice helps to consolidate memories and prevent pupils from forgetting.

Recording as raw marks

We've seen in Chapters 4 and 5 that one of the problems with recording grades very frequently is it forces all formative assessments into a summative structure. In order to allow formative assessments to be flexible and responsive, they need to be freed from the restrictions imposed by grades. However, if we can't record formative assessments through grades or subgrades, what can we record them with?

One possibility is to simply stop recording formative assessment. After all, the aim of formative assessments is to be responsive, and recording these kinds of flexible tasks is hard. There is definitely something to be said for this: capturing and recording every formative assessment would be impossible, because so much of it is ephemeral, and recording no formative assessments at all would be better than measuring them with grades.

Still, recording some types of formative assessment adds a lot to our understanding of how pupils progress. One simple low-tech method is to give pupils five multiple-choice questions at the end of every lesson, and for them to record their answers and scores in a sheet pasted into the back of their exercise book. Obviously, this does not make it easy for teachers to do class or question-level analyses of the type outlined earlier.

A higher-tech solution is to get pupils to answer the questions on tablets and to use software which tracks and analyses their scores over time. An advantage of this is that homework questions could also be easily analysed. We'll investigate how a system like this could work in the final chapter.

One problem we saw in Chapter 5 is that recording raw marks can be misleading; unless we know how difficult the questions were, the raw marks mean very little. A raw mark of 6 out of 10 on one test might be equivalent to a raw mark of 8 out of 10 on another test; working out the relative difficulty of different tests is not straightforward.

Whilst these issues are crucial when creating summative grades, they do not matter as much for formative assessments, for two reasons. First, we are not trying to derive a shared meaning, or a grade, from such questions. It doesn't matter if these questions have a meaning for the class teacher that is not completely shared by anyone else, because the main aim of the question is not to create a shared meaning but for the teacher to work out what to do next. Recording a raw mark together with question-level detail can help with this.

Second, the aim in setting formative assessments is not to set questions that distinguish between candidates or that sample from a large domain. The aim is to set questions that are closely tied to what is being studied. Given this, we should expect pupils to get high scores on such assessments.

The Expressive Writing programme, for instance, expects pupils to get all the formative assessments correct. When they do not, the teacher immediately reteaches the particular concept until pupils do get it right. The assessments are so closely intertwined with the content that it is very easy for pupils to get all the questions right. As a result, one common complaint of teachers teaching the programme is that it is 'too easy'.[19]

However, the programme is designed to be like this: the aim is to teach to mastery. It is based on many of the principles outlined earlier about repetition and spaced practice. When pupils get lots of questions right, this gives the teacher useful feedback and also helps the pupils to build a firm long-term memory of the concept being taught. And, as we've seen, sometimes it can be hard to judge if an assessment task really is easy or not. Despite their apparent simplicity, pupils still do slip up on some of the questions in Expressive Writing. However, a teacher can quickly see this and intervene, which stops these simple mistakes turning into bigger problems.

To sum up, formative assessments can be recorded either on paper or digitally as raw marks. The aim is for teachers to teach to mastery, so pupils should be expected to get 90–100% of questions right.

Assessments which are specific, frequent, repetitive and recorded as raw marks will help pupils and teachers to see if learning is happening; in some cases they will even help pupils to learn.

However, even if formative assessments are as useful as this, we still need a way of reliably measuring the extent of learning. The next chapter will consider ways of improving summative assessment.

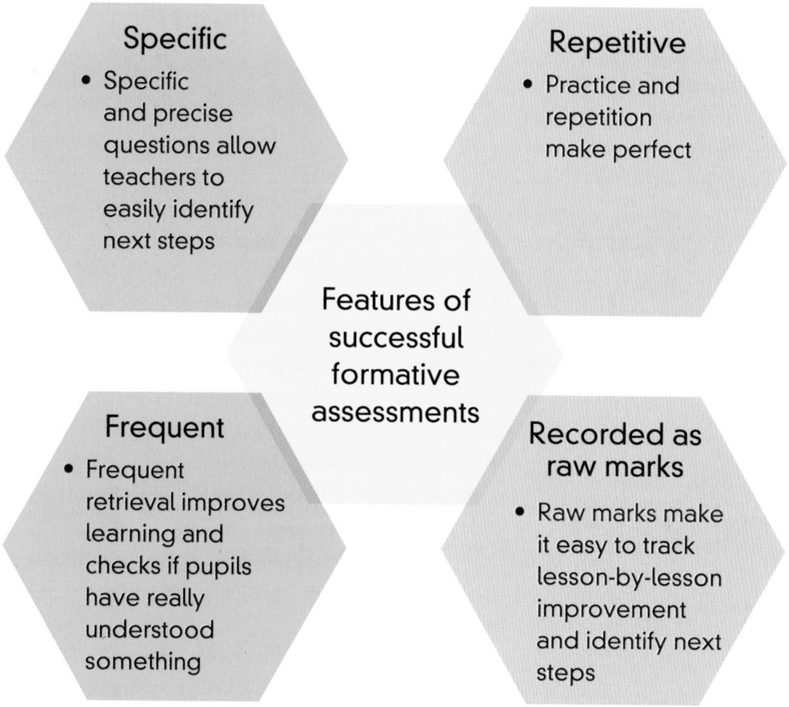

Specific
- Specific and precise questions allow teachers to easily identify next steps

Repetitive
- Practice and repetition make perfect

Features of successful formative assessments

Frequent
- Frequent retrieval improves learning and checks if pupils have really understood something

Recorded as raw marks
- Raw marks make it easy to track lesson-by-lesson improvement and identify next steps

Figure 7.1: Features of successful formative assessments: identifying consequences

Notes

1   British Columbia Ministry of Education, June 2004. *History 12 Resource A Exam Booklet*, p.8

2   See, for example: Driver, R et al. eds., 2005. *Making Sense of secondary science: Research into children's ideas*. London: Routledge

3   See, for example: Hart, K.M. et al., 1981. *Children's understanding of mathematics: 11–16*. London: John Murray

4   See, for example: University of Plymouth, Centre for Innovation in Mathematics Teaching (CIMT) <http://www.cimt.org.uk> accessed 6 November 16

5   See, for example: American Association for the Advancement of Science, AAAS Project 2061 Science Assessment Website <http://assessment.aaas.org/pages/home> accessed 6 November 16

6   Oxford University Press Online Resource Centre. *Garner, Ferdinand & Lawson: Introduction to Politics 2e: Chapter 5* <http://global.oup.com/uk/orc/politics/intro/garner2e/01student/mcqs/ch05/> accessed 6 November 16. This question is part of the online materials supplementing the following textbook: Garner, R, Ferdinand, P. and Lawson, S., 2016. *Introduction to politics*. Oxford: Oxford University Press

7   Little, J.L et al., 2012. Multiple-choice tests exonerated, at least of some charges fostering test-induced learning and avoiding test-induced forgetting. *Psychological Science*, 23(11), pp.1337–1344

8   Bjork, E.L, Little, J.L and Storm, B.C, 2014. Multiple-choice testing as a desirable difficulty in the classroom. *Journal of Applied Research in Memory and Cognition*, 3(3), pp.165–170

9   Roediger, H.L and Karpicke, J.D., 2006. The power of testing memory: Basic research and implications for educational practice, *Perspectives on Psychological Science*, 1(3), pp.181–210

10 Kirschner, P. A, Sweller, J. and Clark, R.E., 2006. Why minimal guidance during instruction does not work: an analysis of the failure of constructivist, discovery, problem-based, experiential, and inquiry-based teaching. *Educational Psychologist*, 41, pp.75–86

11 Sweller, J, 1988. Cognitive Load During Problem Solving: Effects on learning. *Cognitive Science*, 12(2), pp.257–285

12 Laufer, B., 1996. The lexical plight in second language reading: Words you don't know, words you think you know, and words you can't guess. In Coady, J. and Huckin, T., eds. *Second Language Vocabulary Acquisition: A Rationale for Pedagogy*. Cambridge: Cambridge University Press, pp.20–34

13 Bjork, E.L and Bjork, R.A, 2011. Making things hard on yourself, but in a good way: Creating desirable difficulties to enhance learning. In Gernsbacher, M.A, Pew, R.W., Hough, L.M. and Pomerantz, J.R eds. *Psychology and the real world: Essays illustrating fundamental contributions to society*, New York: Worth Publishers, pp.56–64

14 Pronin, E., Puccio, P. and Ross, L, 2002. Understanding misunderstanding: Social psychological perspectives. In Gilovich, T., Griffin, D. and Kahneman, D. eds. *Heuristics and biases*. Cambridge: Cambridge University Press, pp.636–665

15 Willingham, D.T., 2003–2004. Why Students Think They Understand—When They Don't. *American Educator*, Winter 2003–2004 <http://www.aft.org/periodical/american-educator/winter-2003-2004/ask-cognitive-scientist> accessed 6 November 2016

16 Willingham, D.T., 2004. Practice Makes Perfect—But Only If You Practice Beyond the Point of Perfection. *American Educator*, Spring 2004 <http://www.aft.org/periodical/american-educator/spring-2004/ask-cognitive-scientist> accessed 6 November 2016

17 Soderstrom, N.C and Bjork, RA, 2013. Learning versus performance. In Dunn, D.S., ed. *Oxford bibliographies online: Psychology*. New York: Oxford University Press

18 Cepeda, N.J. et al., 2006. Distributed practice in verbal recall tasks: A review and quantitative synthesis. *Psychological bulletin*, 132(3), p.354

19 Engelmann, S., 2007. Student-Program Alignment and Teaching to Mastery. *Journal of Direct Instruction*, 7(1), pp.45–66

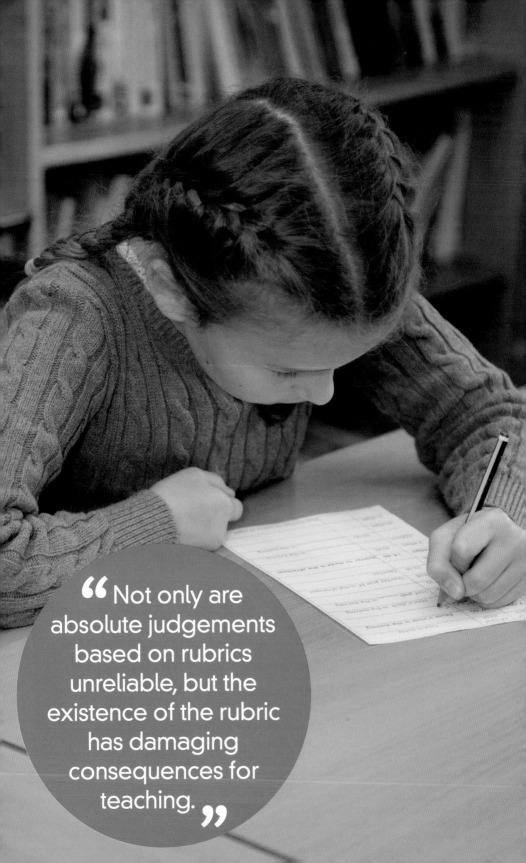

" Not only are absolute judgements based on rubrics unreliable, but the existence of the rubric has damaging consequences for teaching. **"**

Improving summative assessments

8

Even if we design formative assessments perfectly, we still need summative assessments to provide us with a shared meaning of pupil performance and of the relative performance of different curricula and educational approaches. However, as we've seen, the restrictions required by summative assessments often end up distorting formative assessment. So, the aim for summative assessments is for them to provide an accurate shared meaning without becoming the model for every classroom activity.

In previous chapters, we've looked at three ways in which the need for a shared meaning restricts summative assessments. In order to produce a shared meaning, summative assessments have to consist of standard tasks taken in standard conditions, to sample from a large domain of content and to distinguish between pupils. Let's recap each of these briefly now, as well as looking at two other important principles: the need for summative assessments to be taken infrequently, and for them to be reported as a scaled score.

Standard tasks in standard conditions

We've seen already that, for an assessment to produce a shared meaning, it needs to consist of standard tasks taken in standard conditions.

For assessments based on the difficulty model, consisting of a series of questions that get harder and harder, it's easy to see how using standard tasks in standard conditions will result in reliable and comparable scores. A maths paper might require all pupils to answer a series of questions which gradually increase in difficulty. The mark scheme will be clear about what the right answers are, and so there will be a high level of marker reliability.

This is not the case with assessments that are based on the quality model, such as essays or performances. Even if we ask all pupils to do the same essay or performance in the same conditions, marking the task reliably is not as straightforward, because different pupils will have responded to the task in different ways. Indeed, that is what we want: our conception of quality in a piece of creative writing or musical composition allows for, and even welcomes, originality and surprise. However, this does make marking such tasks more difficult. The task needs to encourage originality at the same time as providing a reliable shared meaning.

One way of marking such tasks is to create a rubric which describes the type of quality that is expected at each level and which can be used by markers to judge the quality of each piece of work. However, such rubrics are not particularly good at delivering reliability, and they can even end up compromising the creative and original aspects of the task. The rubrics struggle to deliver reliability for two reasons. First, as we've seen again and again, it's hard to define quality in prose, and prose descriptors can be interpreted in many different ways.[1-2]

Second, judging anything in absolute terms is extremely difficult.[3] An interesting psychological experiment demonstrated this by asking participants to judge the following three items:[4]

(1) Stealing a towel from a hotel

(2) Keeping a dime you find on the ground

(3) Poisoning a barking dog

The participants had to give each action a mark out of 10 depending on how immoral the action was, on a scale where 1 is 'not particularly bad or wrong' and 10 is 'extremely evil'. A second group of participants was asked to do the same, but they were given the following three actions to judge:

(1') Testifying falsely for pay

(2') Using guns on striking workers

(3') Poisoning a barking dog

Item (3) and item (3') are identical, and yet the two groups consistently differ on their ratings of these items. The latter group judge the action to be less evil than the former group. The reason is not hard to see: when you are thinking in terms of stealing towels and dimes, poisoning a barking dog seems heinous. However, in the context of killing humans it seems less so. The implications for marking assessments are clear: a marker who is given a set of essays which are all particularly weak will 'overgrade' the best of the set, and a marker who is given a set of essays which are all particularly strong will 'undergrade' the worst.

Research into marking accuracy has found exactly this problem, along with many other associated distortions and biases.[5] The problem is that our minds are not very good at making absolute judgements. When we are asked to take an action and place it on a scale of 1–10, or to take an essay and match it to a description or grade, we struggle. However, there is one kind of judgement that we are much better at. If we are asked to compare two items or two tasks, we generally give much more reliable and consistent answers; we also find such tasks much less cognitively taxing. Research in this field has therefore led many psychologists to conclude that human judgement is essentially comparative, not absolute.[3]

Not only are absolute judgements based on rubrics unreliable, but the existence of the rubric has damaging consequences for teaching. For example, if a rubric says that in order to get a certain grade, pupils must use fronted adverbials, then teachers will focus on teaching these, and pupils will start to use them. However, pupils may not use a fronted adverbial particularly well or intelligibly. They may write a sentence like: 'Forgettably, he crept through the darkness'. Such a sentence does not really make sense, and the fronted adverbial has been placed there quite mechanically without any real understanding. However, when being marked against a prescriptive mark scheme, an essay that includes such a sentence might end up getting a better mark than one that is more intelligible but does not include a fronted adverbial.

Very prescriptive rubrics end up stereotyping pupils' responses to the task, removing one of the main justifications for such tasks in the first place.[6] Genuinely brilliant and original responses to the task fail because they don't meet the rubric, while responses that have been heavily coached achieve top grades because they tick all the boxes. Worse, these rubrics then effectively encourage this kind of coaching. These unintended consequences were actually anticipated by Polanyi, who argued that if prose descriptors were used in this way, they would 'condemn themselves to absurdity'. In his words:

> *Maxims are rules, the correct application of which is part of the art which they govern. The true maxims of golfing or of poetry increase our insight into golfing or poetry and may even give valuable guidance to golfers and poets; but these maxims would instantly*

condemn themselves to absurdity if they tried to replace the golfer's skill or the poet's art. Maxims cannot be understood, still less applied by anyone not already possessing a good practical knowledge of the art. They derive their interest from our appreciation of the art and cannot themselves either replace or establish that appreciation.

Polanyi, M., *Personal Knowledge*, p.32

This exact problem was seen in primary schools in 2016 in response to a set of primary writing descriptors which are very prescriptive. The primary teacher Michael Tidd has explained the consequences of these descriptors in a way that confirms Polanyi's point:

Recent weeks have been filled not with teachers discussing ideas for great teaching and learning, but with them finding loopholes to hoodwink the moderators and paper over the cracks.

Is there a Year 2 child in the country who hasn't recently completed some work on Little Red Riding Hood? "What good exclamations it contains! All the better for ticking off the standards, my dear."

Suddenly Year 6 teachers, who have bemoaned the influence of films and computer games all year, are encouraging topics about zombies, because the children will be taught the passive voice that way – by zombies, if necessary.

Descriptions abound, not of crimson or scarlet dresses, but now of "rose-like clothing" that provides an opportunity for that all important hyphen. Hyphens are very significant: they feature in the same lists as colons.

Need a few more preposition phrases or adverbial openers? Knock up a quick weather forecast. Lacking evidence of modal verbs? Why not write horoscopes? Indeed, by the end of June, primary children could have written a whole teen magazine.

But what you've really got to watch are the bright pupils – those are the ones most likely to blow your cover. You know those

*avid readers who craft beautiful narratives around clever plots and
subtle metaphors that engage the reader and convey a real sense of
excitement? They are the ones who might not remember that every
good piece of writing needs a dash.*

Tidd, M., Times Educational Supplement, 23 May 2016

What is the solution to such a quandary? Traditionally, one answer
to this problem has involved doing fewer assessments that are based
on the quality model of assessment (thus reducing the need for
judgements based on rubrics), and doing more that are based on the
difficulty model. So, for example, instead of assessing English with an
essay, assess it with multiple-choice questions. This would certainly
give more reliable results, but few people would be happy with exams
that never required pupils to do any extended writing. There is evidence
to show that shorter questions such as multiple-choice can give a valid
inference about pupils' writing skills.[7] But most people would have
legitimate worries about the impact such a change would have on the
curriculum. Multiple-choice questions might be able to give a valid
inference about pupils' writing skills when they are used in a low-stakes
way but if all extended writing was removed from terminal exams,
schools would have less of an incentive to teach such extended writing.
This would obviously be damaging educationally, and it would also
mean that over time, multiple-choice questions would no longer
provide a valid inference about pupils' writing skills.

Using comparative judgement to address problems of rubrics

Given that we need to assess extended writing in terminal exams, is there
any way around the rubric problem? Is it possible to find a method of
assessment which allows us to assess creative and open-ended tasks
reliably and which also allows us to remove the undesirable influence
of the rubric? One approach which has great promise is comparative
judgement.[8-9] Comparative judgement addresses the two problems
of rubrics. First, it does not define quality through prose but through

exemplars. Second, it does not rely on absolute judgements of tasks, but on comparisons.

The quality model of assessment first requires writing prescriptive mark schemes, then training markers in their use and next getting these markers to mark a batch of essays or tasks, before finally bringing them back together to moderate. Instead, comparative judgement simply asks each marker to make a series of judgements about pairs of tasks. Take the example of a piece of creative narrative writing: with comparative judgement, the marker looks at two stories and decides which one is better. Then they look at another pair and decide which one of the two is better, and so on. Each marker makes a series of perhaps 50 or 100 of these judgements which are relatively quick and easy to make. Once the group of markers have made enough decisions, an algorithm is able to combine all those judgements, work out the rank order of all the scripts and associate a mark with each one. The system can also produce GCSE grades or other kinds of national benchmarks if a few pre-graded or example essays are included in the group of scripts to be judged. In some of the early trials which have used comparative judgement, it has delivered levels of reliability in excess of traditional moderation methods.[10-11] It also does not require a rubric. Instead, comparative judgement relies on what Polanyi called 'tacit knowledge'.[12]

This is the kind of knowledge which is very hard to express in words. When markers make a judgement about which of their pair of stories is better, they are using their tacit knowledge about what makes a good story. It is this tacit knowledge which leads to such high levels of reliability on comparative judgement tasks. Different markers all have a similar conception of what quality writing is, even if we cannot precisely define that conception in prose.

One criticism of the comparative judgement process is that, whilst it produces a reliable grade, it offers little in the way of formative feedback to pupils or teachers. At the end of the process, we may know which was the best script out of a group of 100 but we won't know why that was the case. However, in a sense, that is precisely the strength of the comparative judgement model. It separates out the grading process from the formative process. Teachers are therefore free to analyse exactly why it is that a certain task was judged so highly without having to come up with a mechanistic way of deriving a grade from their analysis. In the short term, comparative judgement offers the significant gain of being able to grade essays more reliably and quickly than previously.

But perhaps the more significant longer-term gain it offers is the opportunity to refocus classroom practice away from the rubric and towards more helpful analyses of quality. For example, one extremely useful teaching resource that could be produced through comparative judgement would be a set of annotated exemplar scripts. These would be analogous to the scientific exemplar problems which Kuhn argued are the way that scientific understanding is really communicated.

Imagine if novice teachers could be presented not with a rubric consisting of abstract prose, but with a pack of annotated pupil essays. Something like this was produced as a supplement to APP, but the annotations were linked to the APP statements, and were therefore descriptive, not analytic: the main function of the comments was to justify the grade. To be more useful, the comments should try to explain why certain essays were better than others; the annotations could even provide links to the questions or chapters in the textbook which could help to develop certain aspects of performance. Such a resource would be far more powerful and valuable than a rubric and would lead to far fewer damaging consequences.

Assessments should sample from a large domain of content and distinguish between pupils

Decisions about the difficulty and content of national summative exams are made by national exam boards. However, what about a school that wants to assess summatively more frequently than this? How much content should these assessments cover? How difficult should they be? And, whilst such tasks need to sample from a large domain, to what extent can they be linked to the curriculum being studied in individual schools? Indeed, to what extent can any summative test be designed by teachers in schools, given all the restrictions that apply to it?

One potential solution to these questions is to outsource completely all summative judgements to the kinds of tests provided by external assessment organisations like GL Assessments, the Centre for Evaluation and Monitoring (CEM), and the National Foundation for Educational Research (NFER). These organisations offer assessments that have been nationally standardised and so can give a shared meaning: pupils' scores on them can be compared to those of other pupils nationally.

Whilst many schools appreciate the information they get from these assessments, they do not completely fulfil everything they want from a summative assessment. For example, such tests are only available in English, maths and science. In these subjects, they are fairly remote from the specific curriculum being studied in schools: they broadly assess all the skills included in the national curriculum, but in a fairly generic way and in an order that may be different from that of a school's curriculum. And the tests do not always reflect the types of tasks that pupils have learnt to do in school: for example, few of the tests include any extended writing.

One response to this problem is to use such tests to produce grades on the grounds that they can do it most reliably and not to worry about the fact that they are not closely tied to the school curriculum. After all, it is when we start asking tests to do more than one thing that we start getting problems. Although standardised tests are not closely tied to a school's curriculum, they do draw from the same domains. So, if a school's curriculum is effective, it will lead to improvements on a summative test over time.

Notwithstanding the value of the information from standardised tests, there is still a bit of a gap between these very remote standardised assessments and the very closely tied formative assessments. Is there anything in between these two assessments that could produce a grade but also have a closer link to the school curriculum? For example, an essay or a piece of creative writing in English, or a maths exam with lots of questions that have a range of difficulty, but with a more limited range of topics? Could such tasks provide a grade and a link with the curriculum? It is certainly true that a more curriculum-linked assessment could still be difficult enough and broad enough to produce a shared meaning. However, it is not easy to create such assessments or to interpret the results from them. There are two technical difficulties with creating such assessments and then there is one difficulty with interpreting the results from them, all of which risk distorting the curriculum on which they are based.

Difficulties in creating curriculum-linked assessments

First, it can be hard to tell if the test you have created is difficult enough, or if it has the right spread of difficulty. It can also, as we have discussed before, be difficult to produce reliable grades for school-devised tests that have been taken by small numbers of pupils. One way around this is to compare the results of teacher-devised tests with the results of nationally standardised tests. If the average grade or overall spread of marks in those nationally standardised tests are wildly different from the average grade and spread in the school-devised tests, then it's a sign that the school-devised tests might not have been pitched at the right level. Another possible way around this problem is to use comparative judgement, as described, and collaborate with other schools who have used similar assessments.

Second, such assessments cannot focus solely on what pupils have studied over the most recent term. The content studied over one term is simply not a broad enough domain to sample from. Assessments have to sample from what pupils have learnt in that subject, not just in previous terms but in previous years. Some typical assessments will do this automatically: an unseen reading and writing paper requires pupils to use the vocabulary, background knowledge and writing skills that they have developed throughout their life. Most GCSE papers do this too, although it isn't always clear: the content listed in GCSE specifications is not the only content pupils are tested on. The material in the specification rests on a foundation of other knowledge and skills learnt throughout the pupil's school career.

As a result, interpreting the results of such tests is not easy. These tests are trying to produce a shared meaning and this means they will be relatively insensitive to instruction. But they are also curriculum-linked, which makes it seem as though they should be sensitive to instruction and that pupils should be able to make rapid improvements on them if they have done well in class on that particular topic.

As an example, imagine a pupil in year 7 who arrives at Secondary school with below-average reading and writing skills. The first English unit of study is on *Oliver Twist*. This pupil works hard in class in his first term, receives good teaching and gets good results on all of his formative assessments. The teacher is happy with his classwork. His summative end-of-term assessment is an essay on *Oliver Twist*. This essay is obviously linked to the curriculum the pupils have studied but it is also difficult enough to provide the whole year group with a grade, which means that it requires pupils to apply knowledge and skills that they have learnt prior to that term's instruction. Even though that pupil has done as well as could be expected in class for that term, the assessment will give him a grade that is based on a lot more than that. However, because the assessment was linked to the curriculum, this fact can be obscured: it's easier for teachers and pupils to think that it represents a statement about their performance on the material studied that term. If pupils and teachers do start to think that, the risk is that they interpret a low grade on that assessment as being a reflection on their teaching, learning or curriculum for that term. And the risk then is that they change their approach in order to produce improvements in a grade, but, as we've seen, the methods that can deliver improvements in grades over the short term are ones that involve a focus on short-term performance rather than long-term learning.

A summative assessment can be linked to the curriculum and the most recent unit of study. However, if a grade is awarded, it will not be based solely on that unit and cannot be seen as only reflecting performance on that unit. A pupil may have made great strides in mastering the material in that curriculum unit, but it will not be reflected on the assessment because summative assessments are simply not sensitive enough to measure improvement on smaller units of work.

It is possible, therefore, for teachers to devise their own summative assessments; indeed, in many subjects, if they want a summative grade outside the exam years they have little choice. But there are risks associated with such an approach which have to be carefully managed. One way of managing such risks is to use such assessments less frequently than is currently the case. This is the issue we will look at next.

Infrequency

In previous chapters, we've seen research that suggests most schools grade pupils at least three times a year. We've also seen that the descriptor-based model can lead to the language of grades being used in almost every lesson. What is the ideal frequency for a summative and graded assessment? The answer to this involves a similar logic to the discussion about the right difficulty of an exam.

Summative assessments need to be far enough apart that pupils have the chance to improve on them meaningfully. However, on the large domains of content which most summative exams sample from, pupils will not make particularly rapid improvements. Therefore, once again, if summative assessments are used too frequently, there are risks: either pupils and teachers get demoralised because hard work in class is not showing up as improvement, or pupils and teachers start to focus on short-term tactics which will lead to improvement on the summative exams but will not lead to real improvement in learning. It's because of this that many assessment organisations recommend that many of their tests are taken no more than once or twice a year.[13]

Scaled score

Finally, what is the best way to measure and report summative assessments? Currently, they are often reported as grades such as 'A', 'B' and 'C', or descriptive statements like 'emerging' or 'exceeding'. We've also seen that attempting to break down a grade into raw marks is flawed, because the raw marks needed to achieve a certain standard fluctuate depending on the particular assessment and the version of the assessment being taken. However, there is a scale that does sit underneath grades: the scaled score. A scaled score is the method used for transforming raw marks, which are not comparable, into a scale that is comparable.[14] We saw in Chapter 3 that a typical scaled score used by many assessment organisations is one that has 100 as the average mark, and which runs from approximately 60 to 140. Scaled scores have advantages over raw marks and grades. Unlike raw marks, scaled scores are comparable; unlike grades, they offer finer detail about performance. This finer detail prevents certain distortions from taking place. Some of these distortions caused by grades are significant, and, as Koretz argues, 'create highly undesirable incentives for teachers', so it is worthwhile investigating them a bit further.[14]

Grades suggest that pupil performance falls into categories: that there is a discrete A-grade category, for example, which is distinctive and separate from the B-grade category. When such grades are given labels, not just letters, this is even more the case. A pupil who is categorised as being 'emerging' sounds as though they must be decisively different from a pupil who is categorised as 'expected'; words like 'emerging' and 'expected' 'have their own meanings independent of their use with the standards, and these clearly influence how people interpret the results they are given.'[14] However, in actual fact, pupil performance is continuous, not discrete. Grades and labels 'simply get layered on top of the scale.'[14] They are arbitrary lines placed on top of a continuous distribution. Take a look at Figure 8.1, which shows the proportion of pupils achieving particular scaled scores on a test. The distribution of the scores has produced a smooth and continuous line. Grade boundaries have been placed on top of this distribution, dividing pupils into three categories: 'working towards', 'working at', and 'working in greater depth'.

Pupil A and Pupil C have been given the same grade: they are 'working towards'. However, as we can see from the graph, they are at opposite ends of the 'working towards' category. Pupil A's score is much closer to Pupil B's. However, because their scores on the test fall either side of a grade threshold, they have both been given different grades. Pupil A is 'working towards'; Pupil B is 'working at'. So, Pupils A and C have been

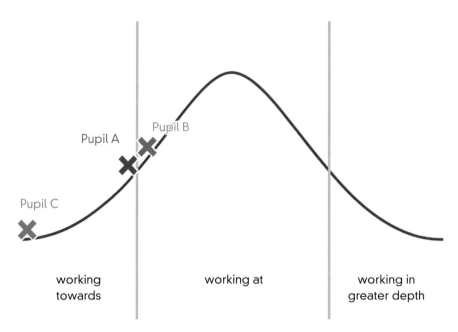

Figure 8.1: A graph which shows that pupil performance is continuous, not discrete

given the same grade, and Pupil B has a different grade, but Pupil A has far more in common with Pupil B than with Pupil C.

Grading systems like this can therefore mislead us about the performance of individual pupils. They can also lead to a further misconception: if we think that pupil performance does come in graded categories, then we are more likely to prioritise moving a pupil from one category to another. This is distorting and damaging, because it means that we will focus more attention on pupils just below a certain threshold, and that we will give more credit to small and statistically insignificant improvements just below a threshold than to big and significant improvements in the middle of a grade.

This problem is another one that has been seen in many schools over the past decade or so, and it has been exacerbated by the existence of accountability targets which measure the success of schools by the number of pupils reaching just one threshold: for example, the percentage of pupils achieving a level 4 or a grade C.[15] To avoid these kinds of distortions, we can record the results of individual pupils' summative assessments as scaled scores; instead of looking at the results of a group of pupils in terms of the percentage achieving a certain mark, we can look at the group average score instead. That way, improvements made by all pupils are included and improvements made at certain arbitrary points are not given a disproportionate weighting.

Of course, this is one area where national systems really do make a big difference. If national exams are recorded as grades, as GCSEs are, then a school might want to use grades instead of scaled scores because these will be easier to understand for parents and pupils. Similarly, if the national accountability system is based on thresholds, as it is at primary, then a school may feel obliged to report its internal assessment data in the same way, even though they recognise the distortions it causes.[16]

One other argument against scaled scores is that it can be hard to get them: teachers cannot create their own tests that produce a scaled score without an awful lot of work. However, they can use the scaled scores from standardised assessments and from comparative judgement, and they can also compare information from their own tests and standardised tests to try and get a rough idea of how difficult their own tests are: for example, a teacher could compare marks on tests to see if the median mark on a standardised test correlates with a particular raw mark on a teacher-created test. Even if it isn't possible for a school to record all of its assessments as scaled scores, using them sometimes and having some idea of the distortions of other methods will still be helpful.

We have now looked at the importance of an accurate model of progression as well as specific improvements in formative and summative assessments. Is there any way all of these principles could be combined into one system? That is what we will consider in the final chapter.

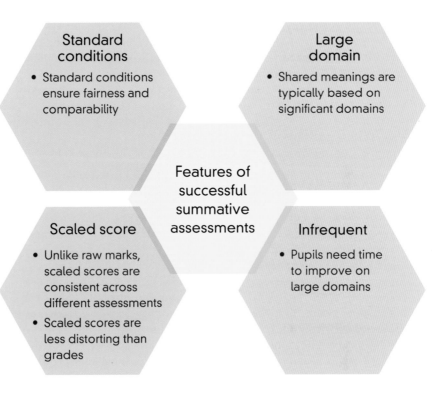

Figure 8.2: Features of successful summative assessments: creating a shared meaning

Notes

1 Polanyi, M., 2012. *Personal Knowledge*. Abingdon: Routledge

2 Kuhn, T.S., 2012. *The Structure of Scientific Revolutions*. Chicago: University of Chicago Press

3 Laming, D., 2003. *Human Judgment: The Eye of the Beholder*. Andover: Cengage Learning EMEA

4 Mozer, M.C. et al., 2010. Decontaminating Human Judgments by Removing Sequential Dependencies. *Advances in Neural Information Processing Systems*, 23

5 For example, see Tisi, J., Whitehouse, G., Maughan, S. and Burdett, N., 2013. *A Review of Literature on Marking Reliability Research* (Report for Ofqual). Slough: NFER, pp.65–67

6 Wiliam, D., 1994. Assessing authentic tasks: alternatives to mark-schemes. *Nordic Studies in Mathematics Education*, 2(1), pp.48–68

7 Hirsch Jr., E.D., 2010. *The Schools We Need: And Why We Don't Have Them*. New York: Anchor, pp.187–204

8 Thurstone, LL., 1927. A law of comparative judgment. *Psychological Review*, 34(4), pp.273–286

9 Pollitt, A., 2012. Comparative judgement for assessment. *International Journal of Technology and Design Education*, 22(2), pp.157–170

10 Jones, I., Swan, M. and Pollitt, M., 2015. Assessing Mathematical Problem Solving Using Comparative Judgement. *International Journal of Science and Mathematics Education*, 13(1), pp.151–177

11 Ofqual, 2015. *A Comparison of Expected Difficulty, Actual Difficulty and Assessment of Problem Solving across GCSE Maths Sample Assessment Materials*

12 Polanyi, M., 1966. *The Tacit Dimension*. Chicago: University of Chicago Press

13 For example: Centre for Evaluation and Monitoring, *Getting the Measure of Primary* <http://www.cem.org/attachments/Getting%20the%20measure%20of%20primary%20-%20brochure%201407.2014.pdf> accessed 6 November 2016; GL Assessment, *Progress Test in English* <http://www.gl-assessment.co.uk/products/progress-test-english> accessed 6 November 2016

14 Koretz, D., 2008. *Measuring Up.* Cambridge, Massachusetts: Harvard University Press, pp.201, 183, 193, 207

15 Compare, for example, the distribution of marks at GCSE in England, where schools are accountable for getting C-grades, and Wales, where schools are not: Cook, C., 2012. English GCSE and Ofqual. *Financial Times,* November 2 <http://blogs.ft.com/ftdata/2012/11/02/english-gcse-and-ofqual/> accessed 6 November 2016

16 Department for Education, 2016. *Primary school accountability in 2016,* p.6 <https://www.gov.uk/government/uploads/system/uploads/attachment_data/file/549568/Primary_school_accountability_in_2016.pdf> accessed 6 November 2016

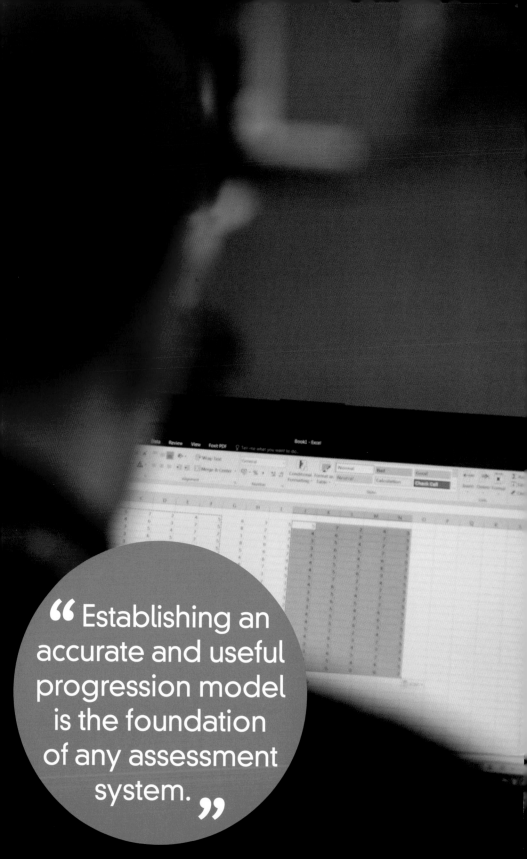

"Establishing an accurate and useful progression model is the foundation of any assessment system."

An integrated assessment system

9

In this final chapter, we'll consider ways in which the improvements put forward in the previous chapters could be integrated into one assessment system.

Progression model

As we've seen all along, establishing an accurate and useful progression model is the foundation of any assessment system, because it explains how pupils make progress and what steps they need to take to get from one stage to the next. The curriculum, the schemes of work, lesson plans and resources can be built on the progression model. The most effective way of bringing all these resources together would be with a textbook.

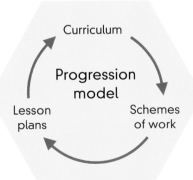

Figure 9.1 Part 1: An integrated assessment system

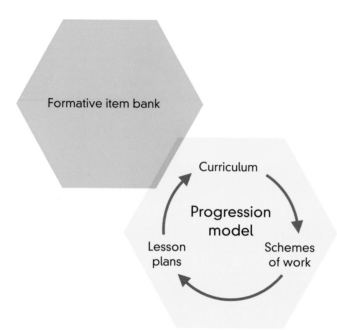

Figure 9.1 Part 2: An integrated assessment system

Formative item bank

This bank is a collection of formative questions which match up to the topics in the curriculum. This bank would be online so that pupils could access it at school or at home. At the end of every chapter or lesson in the textbook, teachers could assign pupils a series of formative questions. Some of these questions would be on the topics pupils had just studied, whilst others would be taken from previous areas of study. The results of these assessments would be recorded on a dashboard that both pupils and teachers would be able to access. This would allow teachers to carry out question- and pupil-level analysis of these assessments, which would then contribute to their planning. If they wanted, they could repeat material from the textbook, or set extra follow-up assessments for certain pupils. Indeed, this bank could automate some of this process: if a pupil got a certain question wrong, it could direct them to a video or worksheet within the textbook addressing that specific question, and then set a series of follow-up questions on the same topic.

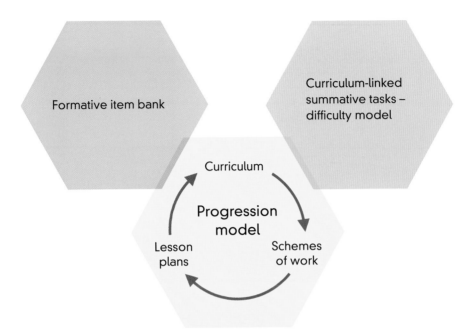

Figure 9.1 Part 3: An integrated assessment system

Summative item bank – difficulty model

This item bank would consist of difficulty-model questions. It would be similar to the formative item bank, except that the items within it would be organised in such a way that it would be possible to use them to get a grade. There would be a couple of ways of doing this. Either the items could be organised into exam papers like those in national exams, which teachers could print off and give to their pupils, or pupils could take the exam digitally, which would allow for it to be 'computer-adaptive'. Computer-adaptive tests adjust the questions each pupil gets based on their response to previous questions, making the tests shorter and the grades they award more accurate. This bank would allow pupils to receive accurate grades in years where there are no national examinations. It could also include past papers and sample papers from exam boards. Theoretically, it would also be possible to store a pupil's final national-exam result and answer scripts in this system; this would allow for a complete overview of their progress over time.

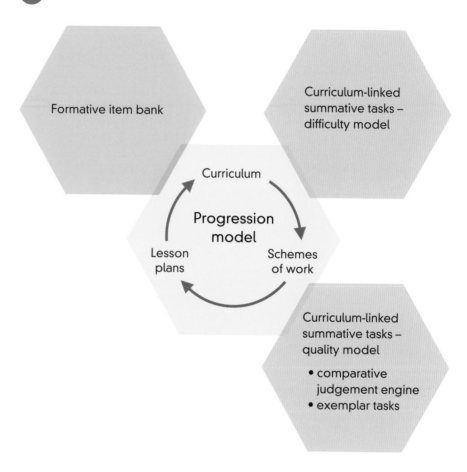

Figure 9.1 Part 4: An integrated assessment system

Summative item bank – quality model

Another similar collection of curriculum-linked summative tasks would be available, based on the quality model of assessment. This element would therefore include a comparative judgement engine so that teachers would be able to upload their pupils' work, add in exemplar work completed by pupils nationally, and then set up a series of judgements they could complete with their colleagues.

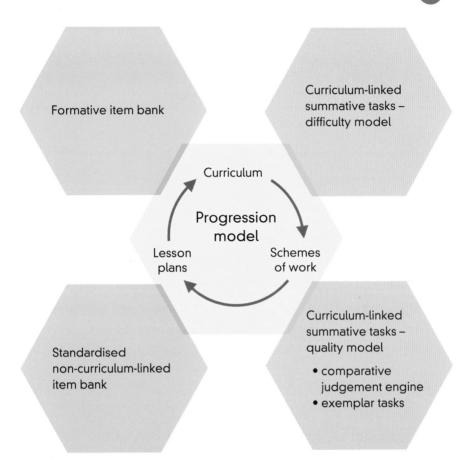

Figure 9.1 Part 5: An integrated assessment system

Standardised task bank

Finally, this bank would consist of standardised and non-curriculum-linked items. This would be made up of the kind of questions currently used in developed ability tests and reading-age tests produced by organisations like GL Assessment and the Centre for Evaluation and Monitoring (CEM). Just as they do now, such tests would provide teachers with information about how their pupils compare to their peer group on some important academic measures. The data from these kinds of tests can prove helpful in setting targets and diagnosing weaknesses.

This bank, unlike the others, is not tied to the curriculum or lessons pupils have been taking; this makes it particularly useful for assessing pupils when they start at a new school and teachers are not sure of the exact curriculum they have studied in the past.

Benefits

Such a system would offer the following benefits:

Coherence

This system would offer the kind of curriculum coherence we looked at in Chapter 6. It would be built on a progression model: a clear understanding of how to progress from novice to expert level in different subjects. Every individual lesson and assessment would have a place as a part of a wider whole; it would be clear to teachers and pupils why certain activities were included, and how everything built towards the final aims.

Pupil ownership

This system would help give pupils some ownership of the curriculum. They would be able to see their progress through the curriculum from the results of the tests they had completed as well as from collections of their work. They would be able to take extra tests from the formative item bank if they wanted, and the formative item bank could adapt to suggest activities that responded to their individual strengths and weaknesses. It would also be possible to build in an element of 'gamification': for example, pupils could collect badges or points for answering questions.

Self-improving

A system like this would produce a lot of data which could be used to investigate links between the different elements. For example, if half the pupils in a class struggled after the first lesson on simultaneous equations but the other half didn't, it would be possible to see if there were any other features that the weaker group had in common: was there a previous topic they had not spent as much time on? It would also be possible to carry out analysis like this across subjects, which is currently very hard to do. For example, if a pupil struggles with their first lesson on molar mass in chemistry, are there previous maths lessons on measurement that they have also struggled with, and might a refresher on this topic help them to progress? Many university professors are already using this approach. Professor Andrew Ng, a computer scientist and a cofounder of Coursera, an online learning company, uses this approach to see how his students are progressing through online content:

> *For example, in tracking the sequence of video lessons that students see, a puzzling anomaly surfaced. A large fraction of students would progress in order, but after a few weeks of class, around lesson 7, they'd return to lesson 3. Why?*
>
> *He investigated a bit further and saw that lesson 7 asked students to write a formula in linear algebra. Lesson 3 was a refresher class on math. Clearly a lot of students weren't confident in their math skills. So Professor Ng knew to modify his class so it could offer more math review at precisely those points when students tend to get discouraged – points that the data alerted him to.*
>
> Mayer-Schönberger, V. and Cukier, K., *Learning with Big Data*, pp.2–3

In subjects where there is less research about models of progression, the data produced by this system could help develop such a model. It would be possible to test various hypotheses about the type of prior knowledge necessary to perform well on certain tasks.

Could this happen?

Every individual element of this system exists already. Products such as Diagnostic Questions and I am Learning have formative item banks where teachers can upload their own questions and use those created by others. GL Assessments and the CEM have standardised item banks for reading tests and developed ability tests. No More Marking offer a free online comparative judgement engine. Exam boards and publishers produce curriculum-linked summative test papers. Schools, the government, publishers and some non-governmental organisations offer progression models, curricula and the resources, lesson plans and textbooks that accompany them.

None of these organisations individually could pull together all of these parts into a whole. For this to happen, it would require unprecedented collaboration between very different organisations. Textbooks would have to follow a progression model, not an exam specification; item-banks would have to match up precisely to textbook content; and schools would have to commit to teaching all this material. It's unrealistic to expect this to happen in the short term. But in the longer term, a system like this could help to solve many of the difficult assessment problems we face.

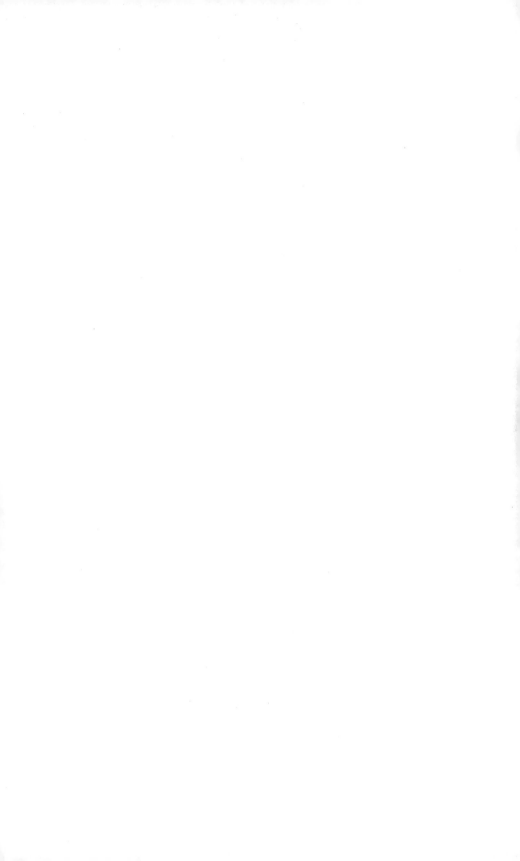

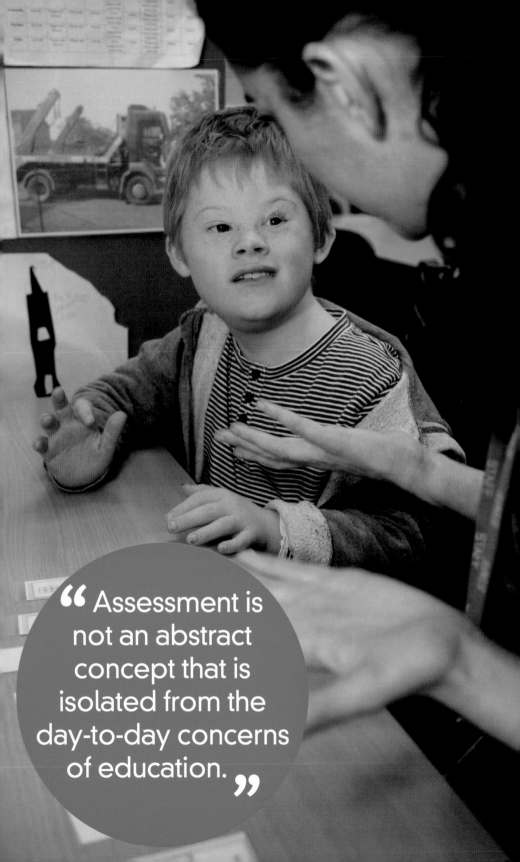

" Assessment is not an abstract concept that is isolated from the day-to-day concerns of education. "

Conclusion

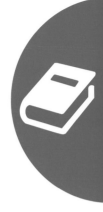

I began this book with two questions: what are the differences between an education that is based only on exam success, and one that is based on developing enduring knowledge and skills? And, more practically, what does an effective and evidence-based school assessment system look like, and how can we avoid the flaws of previous systems? Let's revisit these two questions now.

Exams and education

Exams only sample from wider domains; they are not direct measures of the domain. Because of this, exam success is not the end goal of education, but an indirect measure of the end goal of education. Indirect measures are easily distorted and corrupted, so we have to be careful in the way we use exams and the way we prepare for them. Simplistic backwards planning from past papers, or even from exam specifications, will not deliver the end results we really want. We have to start with our actual goals, not the indirect measures for them.

Counterintuitively, we have also seen that when we do start to use exam activities in class, and to plan backwards from exam papers, this ends with fundamental knowledge being neglected, not emphasised. Excessive exam preparation is not the same as teaching a knowledge-based curriculum; in fact, it is almost the opposite. Exams rightly focus on complex skills and tasks, but these complex skills depend on a hidden body of knowledge. Focussing solely on exam tasks means this hidden knowledge stays hidden, and pupils can only ever develop skills in a superficial and limited way.

Creating an effective assessment system

For an assessment system to help support good teaching, not impede it, we need to accept that complex skills can be broken down into smaller pieces. As a result, many formative assessments will not look much like the final summative assessment and will not be able to be measured on the same scale. The foundation for any assessment system is therefore the model of progression, which makes clear not just the starting point and the end goal but the steps along the way. These models of progression need to be specific to each subject because skills are specific, and do not transfer across subjects as easily as we might think.

Why we should bother with assessment

Assessment can seem like a dry and boring topic, one that is removed from the joy of education and even inimical to it. What I hope I have shown in this book is that the concerns of assessment are central to the wider concerns of education. We can see a similar pattern elsewhere: assessment is essentially a form of measurement, and better measurement has transformed science, medicine, timekeeping, economics and many other fields.[1–2]

Better educational measurement could be similarly transformative. Assessment is not an abstract concept that is isolated from the day-to-day concerns of education. Indeed, as I hope I have shown in this book, flawed ideas about assessment have encouraged flawed classroom practice. Improving assessment and education is a joint project; a project that requires us to reconsider some of our fundamental beliefs about how pupils learn, and one where the potential rewards are similarly far-reaching.

Notes

1 Chang, H., 2004. *Inventing Temperature: Measurement and Scientific Progress.* Oxford: Oxford University Press

2 Allen, D.W., 2011. *The Institutional Revolution: Measurement and the Economic Emergence of the Modern World.* Chicago: University of Chicago Press

Glossary

A level General Certificate of Education (GCE) Advanced Level – exams taken at ages 17–18 in England and Wales

AF Assessment Focus

AfL Assessment for Learning

APP Assessing Pupils' Progress

AQA Assessment and Qualification Alliance

CEM Centre for Evaluation and Monitoring

DfE Department for Education

DCSF Department for Children, Schools and Families (replaced by the Department for Education in 2010)

GCSE General Certificate of Secondary Education

Key Stage Schooling in England and Wales is split into Key Stages.
Key Stage 1 is ages 5–7 (years 1 and 2)
Key Stage 2 is ages 7–11 (years 3, 4, 5 and 6)
Key Stage 3 is ages 11–14 (years 7, 8 and 9)
Key Stage 4 is ages 14–16 (years 10 and 11)

KPI Key Performance Indicator

NAHT National Association of Head Teachers

National Curriculum The current National Curriculum in England was published in 2013 and became statutory in 2015. Academies, free schools and independent schools do not have to follow the National Curriculum.

NFER National Foundation for Educational Research

NGRT New Group Reading Test

OECD Organisation for Economic Co-operation and Development

Ofsted Office for Standards in Education, Children's Services and Skills

PISA Programme for International Student Assessment

RSA Royal Society for the Encouragement of Arts, Manufactures and Commerce

QCDA Qualifications and Curriculum Development Authority

SATs A series of national curriculum tests in England and Wales, colloquialy known as SATs (from the original intention to call them Standard Attainment Tests)

TALIS Teaching and Learning International Survey

TES Times Educational Supplement

WJEC Welsh Joint Education Committee

Bibliography

Ahmed, A. and Pollitt, A, 2010. The Support Model for Interactive Assessment. *Assessment in Education: Principles, Policy & Practice,* 17(2), pp.133–167

AQA, November 2014. *GCSE English/English Language. ENG1H – Understanding and producing non-fiction texts. Report on the Examination* <http://filestore.aqa.org.uk/subjects/AQA-ENG1H-WRE-NOV14.PDF> accessed 6 November 2016

Babbage, C., 2011. *Passages from the Life of a Philosopher.* Cambridge: Cambridge University Press

Bjork, E.L and Bjork, R.A, 2011. Making things hard on yourself, but in a good way: Creating desirable difficulties to enhance learning. In Gernsbacher, M.A, Pew, R.W., Hough, L.M. and Pomerantz, J.R eds. *Psychology and the real world: Essays illustrating fundamental contributions to society,* New York: Worth Publishers, pp.56–64

Boyle, H., 2006. *Opening Minds: A competency-based curriculum for the twenty first century. National Teacher Research Panel* <www.ntrp.org.uk/sites/all/documents/HBSummary.pdf> accessed 19 August 2016

Claxton, G, 2013. *Learning to learn: A key goal in a 21st century curriculum* <escalate.ac.uk/downloads/2990.pdf> accessed 6 November 2016

Coe, R, 2013. *Improving Education: A triumph of hope over experience.* Durham: Centre for Evaluation and Monitoring, Durham University

Department for Children, Schools and Families (known since 2010 as the Department for Education). *The National Strategies: APP Reading: Assessment Focuses and Criteria* <http://webarchive.nationalarchives. gov.uk/20110809101133/http://wsassets.s3.amazonaws.com/ws/nso/pdf/44c1317f5bdb02732731cdf2820f45bb.pdf> accessed 6 November 2016

Department for Children, Schools and Families (known since 2010 as the Department for Education), **2008.** *Assessing pupils' progress in English at Key Stage 3: Teachers' handbook* <http://webarchive.nationalarchives. gov.uk/20130401151715/http://www.education.gov.uk/publications/ eOrderingDownload/sec_eng_app_hndbk.pdf> accessed 6 November 2016

Ericsson, K.A., Krampe, R.T. and Tesch-Römer, C., 1993. The Role of Deliberate Practice in the Acquisition of Expert Performance. *Psychological Review,* 100, pp.363–406

Garner, R., Ferdinand, P. and Lawson, S., **2016.** *Introduction to Politics.* Oxford: Oxford University Press

GL Assessment, 2013. *A Short Guide to Standardised Tests* <http://www. gl-assessment.co.uk/sites/gl/files/images/Guide-to-Standardised-Tests. pdf> accessed 6 November 2016

Green, J. Question level analysis in science. *the science teacher* <http:// thescienceteacher.co.uk/question-level-analysis/>

Hattie, J., 2009. *Visible Learning: A Synthesis of Over 800 Meta-Analyses Relating to Achievement.* New York, Routledge

Hertfordshire Grid for Learning, 2009. *Student-Friendly APP Reading Assessment Focuses* <http://thegrid.org.uk/learning/english/ks3-4-5/ks3/ assessment/index.shtml#app> accessed 6 November 2016

Hirsch Jr., E. D., **1987.** *Cultural Literacy: What Every American Needs to Know.* Boston: Houghton Mifflin

Kirschner, P.A., Sweller, J. and Clark, R.E., **2006.** Why Minimal Guidance During Instruction Does Not Work: An Analysis of the Failure of Constructivist, Discovery, Problem-Based, Experiential, and Inquiry-Based Teaching. *Educational Psychologist,* 41, pp.75–86

Koretz, D., **1998.** Large-scale Portfolio Assessments in the US: evidence pertaining to the quality of measurement. *Assessment in Education: Principles, Policy & Practice,* 5(3), pp.309–334

Koretz, D., **2008.** *Measuring Up.* Cambridge, Massachusetts: Harvard University Press

Kuhn, T.S, 2011. Second Thoughts on Paradigms. In *The Essential Tension: Selected Studies in Scientific Tradition and Change.* Chicago: University of Chicago Press, pp.293–320

Larkin, J., McDermott, J., Simon, D.P. and Simon, H.A, 1980. Expert and novice performance in solving physics problems. *Science,* 208(4450), pp.1335–1342

Mayer-Schönberger, V. and Cukier, K, 2014. *Learning with Big Data: The Future of Education.* Boston: Houghton Mifflin Harcourt

Oates, T., 2010. *Could do better: Using international comparisons to refine the National Curriculum in England.* Cambridge: University of Cambridge Local Examinations Syndicate <http://www.cambridgeassessment.org. uk/images/112281-could-do-better-using-international-comparisons-to-refine-the-national-curriculum-in-england.pdf> accessed 20 August 2016

Oates, T., 2014. *Why textbooks count: A policy paper.* Cambridge: University of Cambridge Local Examinations Syndicate

Ofsted, 2008. *Curriculum innovation in schools* <http://www. readyunlimited.com/wp-content/uploads/2015/09/Curriculum-Innovation-in-schools-ofsted.pdf> accessed 19 August 2016

Ofsted, 2011. *Successful science: An evaluation of science education in England 2007–2010.* <www.ofsted.gov.uk/resources/successful-science> accessed 19 August 2016

Ofsted, 2012. *Moving English forward: Action to raise standards in English.* <https://www.gov.uk/government/uploads/system/uploads/ attachment_data/file/181204/110118.pdf> accessed 19 August 2016

Polanyi, M., 2012. *Personal Knowledge.* Abingdon: Routledge

Roediger, H.L and Karpicke, J.D., 2006. The power of testing memory: Basic research and implications for educational practice. *Perspectives on Psychological Science,* 1(3), pp.181–210

Rohrer, D. and Taylor, K, 2006. The effects of overlearning and distributed practise on the retention of mathematics knowledge. *Applied Cognitive Psychology,* 20(9), pp.1209–1224

Tidd, M., 2016. Instead of discussing great teaching and learning, we're looking for loopholes to hoodwink the moderators. *Times Educational Supplement*, 23 May <https://www.tes.com/news/school-news/breaking-views/instead-discussing-great-teaching-and-learning-were-looking> accessed 6 November 2016

Welsh Joint Education Committee, Summer 2014. *GCSE Examiners' Reports English, English Language and English Literature (England/Out of Wales)* <http://www.wjec.co.uk/qualifications/english/GCSE%20 English%20Lang%20English%20Lit%20Report%20%28England%29. pdf?language_id=1> accessed 6 November 2016

Welsh Joint Education Committee, November 2013. *GCSE Examiners' Reports English and English Language* <http://www.wjec.co.uk/uploads/ publications/19505.pdf> accessed 6 November 2016

Wiliam, D., 2000. *Integrating formative and summative functions of assessment.* Paper presented to Working Group 10 of the International Congress on Mathematics Education, Makuhari, Tokyo, August 2000

Wiliam, D., 2011. *Embedded formative assessment.* Indiana: Solution Tree Press

Wiliam, D., 2011. *What assessment can—and cannot—do* <http://www.dylanwiliam.org/Dylan_Wiliams_website/Papers_files/ Pedagogiska%20magasinet%20article.docx> accessed 6 November 2016. Originally published in Swedish as 'Bryggan mellan undervisning och lärande' in *Pedagogiska Magasinet*, September 2011.

Wiliam, D., 2014. *Principled Assessment Design.* London: SSAT

Wiliam, D. and Black, P., 1996. Meanings and Consequences: a basis for distinguishing formative and summative functions of assessment? *British Educational Research Journal*, 22(5), pp.537–548

Willingham, D.T., 2007. Critical thinking: Why is it so hard to teach? *American Educator*, Summer 2007. pp.8–19

Willingham, D.T., 2009. *Why Don't Students Like School?* San Francisco: Jossey-Bass

Copyright acknowledgements

We are grateful to the authors and publishers for use of extracts from their titles and in particular for the following:

AQA material is reproduced by permission of AQA

Babbage, Charles: *Passages from the Life of a Philosopher*. Cambridge University Press, 2011.

Bambrick-Santoyo, Paul: 'Driven by data: A practical guide to improve instruction'. John Wiley & Sons, 2010.

Beck, Isabel L, McKeown, Margaret G. & Kucan, L: *Bringing Words to Life: Robust vocabulary instruction*. © 2013 The Guilford Press. Reprinted with permission of Guilford Press.

From Psychology and the Real World: Essays Illustrating Fundamental Contributions to Society 2e by FABBS Foundation and edited by Morton Ann Gernsbacher, et Al. Copyright 2015. All rights reserved. Reprinted by permission of Worths Publishers.

Coe, R: 'Improving Education: A triumph of hope over experience', Centre for Evaluation & Monitoring: Durham University, 2013 from http://www.cem.org/attachments/publications/ImprovingEducation2013.pdf Reproduced by permission of the author.

Extracts reprinted with permission from the Spring 2004 and Summer 2007 issues of *American Educator*, the quarterly journal of the American Federation of Teachers, AFL-CIO.

Extract from Department for Children, Schools and Families, *Assessing pupils' progress in English at Key Stage 3 Teachers' handbook*, http://webarchive.nationalarchives.gov.uk/20130401151715/ http://www.education.gov.uk/publications Contains public sector information licensed under the Open Government Licence v3.0.

Extract from GL Assessment, A Short Guide to Standardised Tests, © 2013 from http://www.gl-assessment.co.uk Reproduced by permission of GL Assessment.

Larkin, J. et al: 'Expert and novice performance in solving physics problems'. Science 208- 1335-1342. Reprinted by permission of Science/AAAS.

Mayer-Schönberger, Viktor, and Cukier, Kenneth: *Learning with big data: The future of education.* Houghton Mifflin Harcourt, 2014. Reproduced by permission.

Oates T: 'Could do better: Using international comparisons to refine the National Curriculum in England' (2010), http://www.cambridgeassessment.org.uk/ images/112281-could-do-better-using-international-comparisons-to-refine-the-national-curriculum-in-england.pdf

Extract from National Teacher Research Panel: Engaging Teacher Expertise. 'Opening Minds: A competency-based curriculum for the twenty first century' (2006), www.ntrp.org.uk/sites/all/documents/HBSummary.pdf
Reproduced by permission.

Extract from Office for Standards in Education, Children's Services and Skills. 'Curriculum innovation in schools' (2008),
http://webarchive.nationalarchives.gov.uk/20141124154759/http://www.ofsted.gov.uk/resources/curriculum-innovation-schools
Contains public sector information licensed under the Open Government Licence v3.0.

Extract from Office for Standards in Education, Children's Services and Skills. 'Successful science: An evaluation of science education in England 2007–2010' (2011), www.gov.uk/government/publications/successful-science-strengthes-and-weaknesses-of-school-science-teaching
Contains public sector information licensed under the Open Government Licence v3.0.

Extract from Office for Standards in Education, Children's Services and Skills. Moving English forward: Action to raise standards in English (2012), www.gov.uk/government/publications/moving-english-forward
Contains public sector information licensed under the Open Government Licence v3.0.

Extract from Welsh Joint Education Committee, GCSE Examiners' Reports English and English Language, November 2013,
http://www.wjec.co.uk/uploads/publications/19505.pdf
Reproduced by permission.

Polanyi, Michael: *Personal knowledge Towards a Post-Critical Philosophy.* © 2015. University of Chicago Press. Reproduced by permission.

Question 14 from 'Edexcel GCSE Mathematics B Unit 1: Statistics and Probability (Calculator)' Tuesday 9 November 2010, © 2010 Edexcel Limited. Reproduced by permission of Pearson UK

Roediger, H L, and Karpicke. J D: "The power of testing memory: Basic research and implications for educational practice." Perspectives on Psychological Science 1.3 (2006): 181-210. Sage Publications.